Essential Oils Collection:
150 Amazing Essential Oils Recipes For Diffusers, Aromatherapy, Skin And Hair Care

Table of content

Introduction

If you have spent any amount of time online, you know that it is important to watch what you are putting in or on your body. You know that there are medications and supplements that are meant to help your health in a variety of ways, but then you read that you should avoid a whole list of items that are then found in the supplements you are using.

So what do you do?

You know that you want to do the best thing for your health and your body, but what are you supposed to do when the very things you are supposed to use for your health end up being full of the very things you try to avoid.

You think of how you want to do what is best for your health, for your family, and for the planet, but you don't think you can do this if you are supporting the synthetic products that are on the shelves today.

This is a common feeling that a lot of people share, and thankfully the number one solution to this problem is also the solution to your health concerns. Essential oils are entirely natural, free of harmful synthetic chemicals, and can be used in more ways than any synthetic medication you could imagine.

You have a headache, you want to relax, and you want to settle the house down at the end of the day.

You don't want to turn to the synthetic medications that are full of warnings and things to watch for, but what do you do?

Essential oils is the answer. You can diffuse a few drops in a diffuser, you can apply a few drops directly to your skin, or you can even add certain kinds to tea, and you get the same great results.

Calm, quiet tranquility fills your home, and you feel better.

That's just the beginning. The more familiar you get with essential oils, the more you will be able to treat the ailments that arise, and the more natural you can live.

So are you ready to jump into the world of essential oils?

Naturally.

Chapter 1 – Getting Started

There is a lot of excitement when you start out in this journey, but before you just dive in and spread oils on everything, I want to get you started on the right track. This means you need to know what you are doing from the beginning.

You can't just toss essential oils around and see what happens, you have to know what each oil does, and how to use them for your particular symptoms. This is something you can use both ways. You can use this knowledge to use the right oil for your particular ailment, and you can avoid the oils that won't help you or potentially make you feel worse.

On the other hand, if you know what oils create different results, you will be able to set up your home with a lot of preventative aspects, meaning you won't get sick as often or feel the stress to begin with.

So, let's dive in and learn the facts about essential oils, how to use them, and what oils work well with each other.

Knowledge is an effective weapon.

The Wonder Oils

While each section you find is going to have its own list of oils, there are a few oils that seem to stand out from the rest. Yes, there are going to be times when you need to treat something specific, and you will need an equally specific oil to get the job done, but on the other hand, you are going to see a few oils show up time and time again, no matter what the ailment happens to be.

These are the oils I would like to refer to as the Wonder Oils, because there are so many ways using these oils can make your life better.

They are good for the specifics, and they are good for the broad categories.

Whether you are dealing with aches, pains, illness, insomnia, or want to promote things such as peace, tranquility, focus, happiness, and better relationships, these are the oils you always want to have on hand.

Peppermint

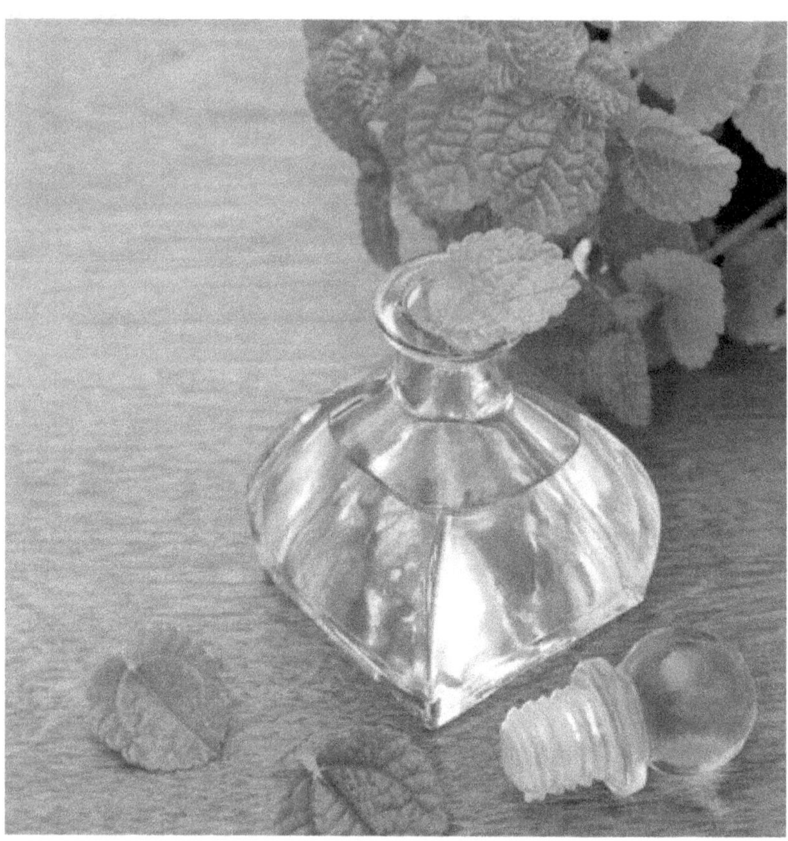

While many of us may associate this scent and taste with the holidays, there are a few things you need to know about this delightful oil that has nothing to do with Christmas trees or Santa Clause.

Peppermint oil has a light, fresh scent that blends exceptionally well with most other oils. It can be diffused for aroma therapy, applied topically on various aches and pains, and it can be enjoyed internally if it is highly diluted in water or tea. This oil is going to ease pains, clear your mind, and make you feel better and at peace.

It is abundantly available... you can purchase it not only online but in a variety of health and wellness stores to even large chain department stores. This oil truly is a wonder worker, and I suggest you keep plenty of it on hand at all times.

Lavender

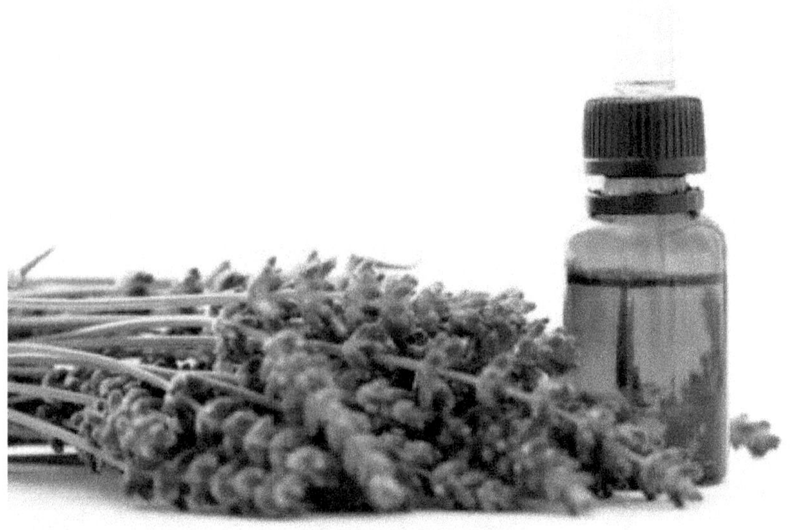

The floral scent of lavender is soothing to the mind, body, and soul. You would be amazed at how many people there are who think they don't like floral scents, but gravitate toward lavender.

Certainly among the best of the best, lavender is easily considered a Wonder Oil.

This oil is like peppermint in regards to the fact it will ease many of your life's ailments. Whether you are tense, stressed, or unable to sleep, a few drops of this oil spread across your forehead, blended into your bath water, or diffused in your bedroom is going to ease all of that tension that has built up and help you not only fall asleep, but stay asleep.

When you realize you can't become dependent on it, but you can use it as freely as you like, you are going to realize even more why you should keep this on hand at all times.

Make a space in your cabinet to house your lavender, peppermint, and tea tree oils, and there are few things you will face that you won't be able to handle.

Tea tree

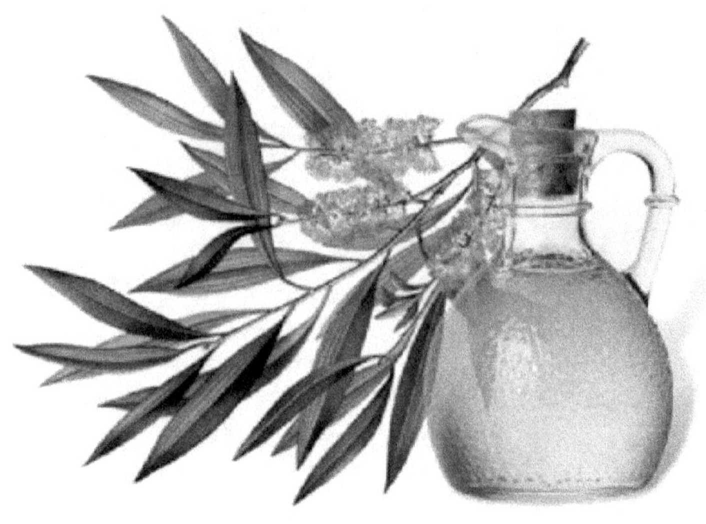

https://www.google.com/search?
q=tea+tree+oil&espv=2&biw=1366&bih=623&source=lnms&tbm=isch&sa=X&ved=0ahUKEwjR2YiQq4LNAhVIM-
FIKHT7rCgkQ_AUIBygC#imgrc=wfzRemDWCYN4oM%3A

When it comes to physical ailments and imperfections, few things are going to do more for you than tea tree oil. While this oil has a strong, somewhat overwhelming scent, the benefits it does for your skin are far beyond the strong scent it holds.

Tea tree oil is a natural antiseptic. You can apply it to scrapes, cuts, and even acne and it will heal and clear up the imperfection. Excellent for hair, skin, and even sore throats and coughs, this oil is best diffused into the air for aroma therapy or mixed with a carrier oil and applied topically.

If you want to lighten the scent of this Wonder Oil, you can blend it with less offensive oils such as lavender, rose, or lemon. Another terrific benefit that comes with tea tree oil is that it is even more abundant than peppermint or lavender. You can purchase large vials of the purest form online or in health food stores, and it doesn't cost nearly as much as some of the more exotic oils do.

This oil's benefits far outweigh the scent, so make sure to get a large vial of it and keep it up in your cabinet along with the lavender and peppermint. You will be so glad you did.

Chapter 2 – The Best of the Blends

You may only be experiencing one feeling, or you may want to promote a singular feeling, in which case you only need to choose the oil or oils that you enjoy. There are going to be times, however, when you need to address more than one problem at a time, or when you want to create a blend of energy in your home.

To do this, you need to combine oils in properly to get the desired effect.

Thankfully, blending oils is not only easy, it is encouraged to create the best fragrances and optimum results, so you won't have any problem at all finding the right blend for your needs.

The trick to getting the best of the blends is to know how to blend the oils yourself

If you get online, you are going to find that there are plenty of blends all ready to go. The supplier puts them together and sells them as a blend, usually under the name of what you need it for.

For example, you can purchase an oil blend from Doterra called "On Guard". It is an immunity support oil, but if you look closer at it, you will see that it is, in fact, a blend of the everyday oils you have on hand such as wild orange, clove bud, cinnamon, eucalyptus, and rosemary.

While there is a lot of convenience to purchasing the oil already blended, you are going to find that you will save a lot of money, and get a lot more of the product if you purchase the oils separately and blend them yourself.

Wait, purchasing all of those oils separately isn't going to be inexpensive... the blend is a lot cheaper to buy as it is

Yes, that may be true, but if you think about it, if you purchase the ingredients separately, not only do you get enough to make the blend yourself, but you also get the extra oils left over to put to other use.

This is going to come in handy if you want to have the immunity support, as well as treat any ailment you already have, or simply to set some aside until you need it again. You see, when you are blending the oils yourself, you always have a lot of each on hand, simply because you only use a few drops of each one when you do use it.

So that brings us to the actual blending aspect.

When you blend the oils yourself, make sure you look at the total number of drops you are going to be using at the end result. If you are making enough to save some, keep the ratios the same, but if you are only mixing one time use at a time, watch out for how much you are actually using.

What this means is that if you are going to use the oils to make the equivalent to Doterra's On Guard, you need to realize that the 2 drops you use from that bottle are 2 blended drops.

I know that sounds confusing at first, but think about it this way. If you are mixing in the On Guard into your tea to sip on, you only need 1 or 2 drops to do it. All of those oils I listed that create this blend come together in those 2 drops you put into your tea.

If you were to take each of those drops and place only 1 drop each in your tea separately, then you will end up with 5 or 6 drops, which is simply too much to ingest at one time. If you put this all in your tea at once, you will run into problems from overdosing on the oils.

To get around this, you need to cut back on the amount of oils you are using in your tea, or (better yet) blend them all separately then take 2 drops of what you have blended. The most important thing you need to remember when it comes to essential oils is that you can overdose, and too much of some of them can be toxic.

Keep small jar glasses on hand, or purchase some of your own vials to store the extra oils you blend. This is going to keep them safe until you need them again, and help you stay on track with the proper dosage of the oils.

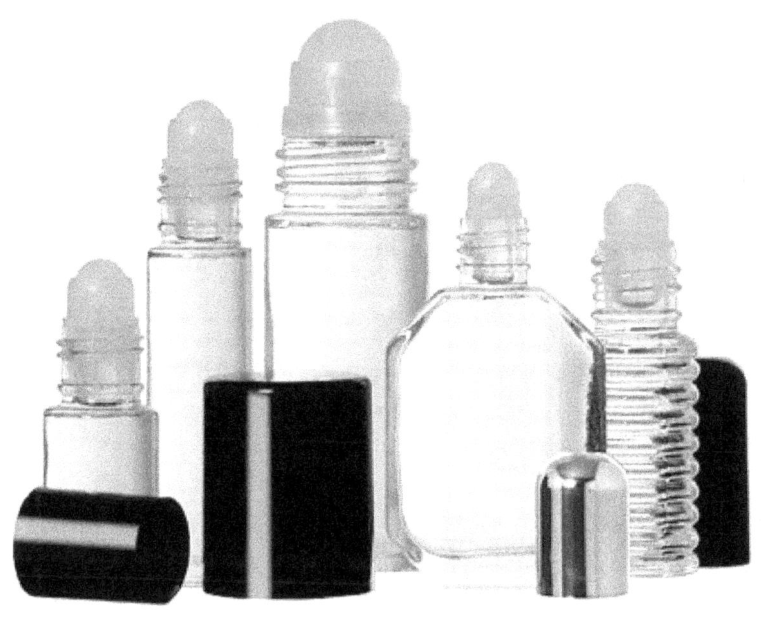

https://www.google.com/search?q=roll+on+bottles&espv=2&biw=1366&bih=623&source=lnms&tbm=isch&sa=X&ved=0ahUKEwirnbWvqoLNAhVHGl-IKHR3CDn8Q_AUIBygC#imgrc=SO6aHKfGslPGZM%3A

Small vials that have the drop lid are available online, or you can even get them locally at a number of stores. One of the major benefits to mixing your own blends in your own bottles is that you get to then choose the bottles you want to use as well.

This means you can create your own mists, roll ons, or drop bottles to suit your own taste, and keep them on hand where you want them. Say you want to take an anti-stress blend to work with you? No problem!

Purchase a roll on dispenser, mix up your favorite blend or just use your favorite anti-stress oil, fill your roll on dispense, and toss it in your purse. No matter where your day goes you will have your instant anti-stress mechanism at just an arm's length away, and your day is going to go so much better.

When you are creating your own blends, start with the desired effect you want your blend to have, and move on from there.

For example, if you want a blend that is going to help you sleep, but you also want to relieve tension and stress besides, start with the lavender. You want there to be more lavender in this blend than anything else, so I would recommend starting with 10 or 12 drops of this oil.

Then, pick the other oils you want. Peppermint is great for stress relief, so choose this one next, but don't put in the same amount. Perhaps 6 or 7 drops to suit your own taste.

What you want to keep in mind is that you want to use the most of your main focus, then add in the secondary oils as secondary benefits. Once you have this down, you can make any blend you want for any use you want.

Get creative!

Chapter 3 – Oils by Symptoms or Desired Effect

There are times when you are looking through the oils to see what they do, but there are also times when you feel a certain way and you want to find the oils that make it better.

What I mean by this is that you may enjoy the smell of rose oil and lavender oil, so you diffuse this in your home often. You are going to gain the amazing benefits that come from diffusing this oil... which means you are going to feel calm, relaxed, open, etc... but this doesn't help when you are suffering from a headache.

So, if you happen to have some sort of ailment (a headache, a stomach ache, a tooth ache), you need to know which oils to use specifically for these problems.

Here are oils separated into categories based on the symptoms you feel.

You can use one of the oils in the category, or you can mix and match as you please to take care of many of your symptoms.

Body Aches and Pains

Body aches and pains are annoying as well as debilitating. When you feel any of these symptoms, you know you want to get better as soon as possible.

I suggest for any of the oils or oil blends you use here, mix a few drops with a carrier oil and massage onto the aching area.

You can also add 10 to 12 drops into a warm bath and soak your pain away.

Headaches

Eucalyptus

Lavender

Peppermint

Stomach aches

Peppermint

Ginger

Roman chamomile

Melissa

Star anise

Grapefruit

Spearmint

Cardamom

Coriander

Fennel

Aniseed

Joint pain and stiffness

Sweet marjoram

Chamomile

Rosemary

Peppermint

Eucalyptus

Muscle cramps

Peppermint

Lemongrass

Basil

Vetiver

Sage

Cypress

Grapefruit

Rosemary

Natural Cold and Flu Remedies

When it comes to treating the cold and flu, I suggest you use a diffuser next to your bed or couch. The oils will fill the air and the aroma therapy will clear the illness right out.

If you are dealing with specific aches such as a sore throat, cough, or headache, you may also mix the oils of your choice with a carrier oil and massage it into the infected area, or add a drop or two to tea and sip on it.

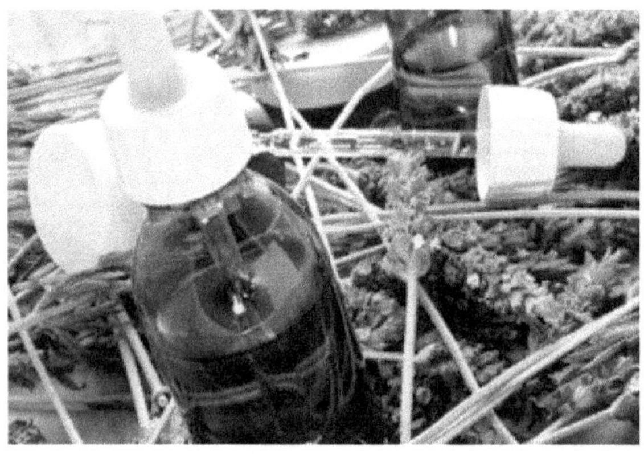

Colds

Lavender

Eucalyptus

Thyme

Rosemary

Garlic

Sandalwood

Lemon

Chamomile

Peppermint

Sore Throat

Eucalyptus

Oregano

Sage

Tea tree

Ginger

Peppermint

Cough

Lavender

Peppermint

Lemongrass

Frankincense

Lemon

Stress

No matter what kind of job you work or what kind of life you live, you are going to deal with a level of stress.

To rid your mind and body of that stress, I strongly suggest you use these oils or any blend of these oils in a diffuser, or add 10 to 12 drops into your hot bath water before you soak in the tub.

Tension

Helichrysum

Peppermint

Spearmint

Roman chamomile

Eucalyptus

Lavender

Insomnia

Lavender

Roman chamomile

Sweet marjoram

Vetiver

Ylang ylang

Anxiety

Basil

Clary sage

Bergamot

Frankincense

Ylang ylang

Marjoram

Peppermint

The Air of the House is the Mood of the Home

They say prevention is the best cure, and if you set up your home to be a safe haven, you are going to skip out on a lot of stressful symptoms that pop up in day to day life.

Use these oils in diffusers around your home. Diffusers aren't expensive and they are easy to maintain.

Prevent ailments and issues and promote peace and health with these oils blended into the air of your home at all times.

The Essentials you will need:

To promote tranquility

Chamomile

Roman chamomile

Lavender

Cedar wood

To promote happiness

Orange

Rose

Jasmine

Ginger

Cloves

Sandalwood

Petitgrain

Frankincense

Lemon

Geranium

To promote energy

Black pepper

Bergamot

Grapefruit

Peppermint

Rosemary

Thyme

Lemon

Basil

Fennel

To promote peace

Tangerine

Orange

Patchouli

Ylang ylang

Cassia

Davana

German chamomile

Cistus

Lavender

Lemon

Chapter 4 – The Practical Side of Things

In life there are far more things we want to address and take care of besides mood and colds. You want beautiful hair, you want to lose weight or maintain a weight loss. Your teenagers want clear skin and you want to avoid or get rid of the wrinkles that somehow appeared around your mouth and eyes.

Sure, it's great to know how to address a headache or sleeplessness, but once you know how to also get rid of such things as acne, wrinkles, and oily hair, you are going to be completely taken care of in your oil usage.

That is why I have included this chapter, so you know exactly what you can use to treat or prevent those physical imperfections you don't want to have to deal with any longer.

And when you combine the fact you get to save money as well as save your skin from harmful chemicals, you have a complete win, and everyone wants to have that.

Essential Skin Care

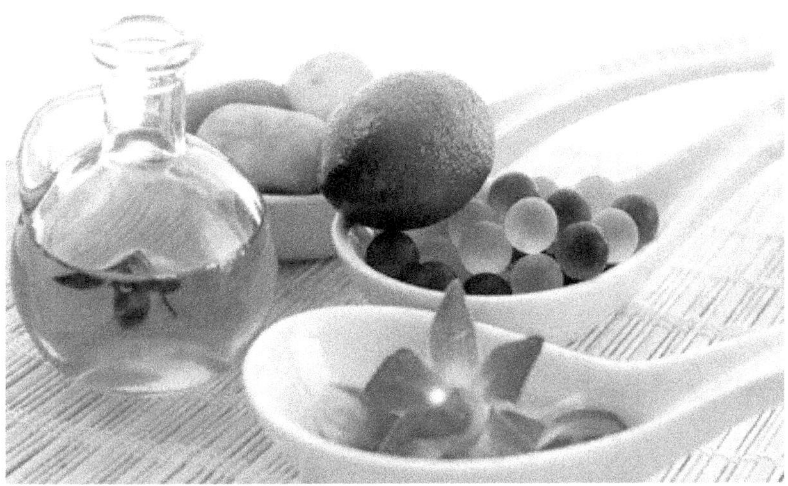

People of all ages across the globe spend hundreds and thousands of dollars each year on various skin care products. Each of the products claim they are going to do the magic trick, but most of them end up not working anyway.

Not to mention these products are full of chemicals you don't want on your skin. Using essential oils are always a better choice, and I promise you that you are going to see better results using these than you ever did with store products.

To use these, mix with your face soap, moisturizer, or with a carrier oil and apply directly to the spot you want to focus on.

How to get rid of acne

Jojoba

Lavender

Tea tree

Orange

Frankincense

Get rid of those wrinkles!

Myrrh

Frankincense

Rose

Carrot seed

Lavender

Geranium

Sandalwood

Minimize the appearance of pores and say goodbye to freckles

Lemon

Tea tree

Lemongrass

Carrot seed

Geranium

Frankincense

For the Hair

Many commercials proudly proclaim that your hair is as unique as you, but you don't find this to be a good thing when you can't find any product that does what you need it to do.

Here are the oils you want to turn to based on what you need for your hair. Blend a few drops in with your shampoo and wash as you normally would.

The results are real, and you are going to love them.

The best oily hair treatment

Lavender

Cedar wood

Peppermint

Frankincense

Sage

Basil

Clary sage

Juniper

Hair growth oils

Thyme

Lavender

Rosemary

Moisture for the dry hair

Clary sage

Lemon

Thyme

Tea tree

Cedar wood

Weight Loss and Weight Management

It seems that majority of people want to lose weight, but once they do, it is a struggle to keep it off. If you bring in these oils, you are going to see the weight melt away, as well as keep it off for good.

I suggest you use a diffuser for these oils, or that you highly dilute a drop or two into a tall glass of water. The results are real, entirely natural, and not even remotely dangerous.

You really can lose that weight for good, and enjoy the results, knowing they are going to last.

Essential weight loss

Lemon

Grapefruit

Cypress

Ginger

Peppermint

Cinnamon

Garlic

Perfect weight management

Grapefruit

Tangerine

Lemon

Spearmint

Ocotea

Cinnamon bark

Thieves

And, of course.... Peppermint

I'm sure you saw the overlap I mentioned in chapter 1 of all the ways you can use the top 3 oils, but I do strongly urge you to go out and get as many oils as you can find. They have dozens for sale on Amazon, or you can look into the other private suppliers that are around both online and locally.

No matter where you decide to get your essential oils, the important thing you need to remember is to check that they are pure. A pure essential oil is going to come in a dark bottle, as this is the best way to store them. The liquid itself is going to be strongly scented, and have an oily appearance just by looking at it.

If you get your oils from reputable sources, you have nothing to worry about, so just go through somewhere you trust, and make sure it says on the label that it is 100% pure before you buy.

Chapter 5 – The Tricks of the Trade: How to Use Essential Oils

You can know all kinds of things about essential oils, whether it be which ones are best for certain symptoms, what blends smell the best, or what kind of oils you want to avoid in various situations, but all of this is just head knowledge unless you know how to take them from the vial and put them into your life.

There are a number of different methods that people use when it comes to essential oils.

The most common are:

1. Diffusing

2. Applying topical

3. Taking internally

Let's take a moment now to look at each one, and you can decide which method you prefer for yourself, or what combination of methods you want to use. Some people choose one, others combine one or two, then there are those that use all three, the great thing about essential oils and knowing how to use them is that you can do what you want, when you want it.

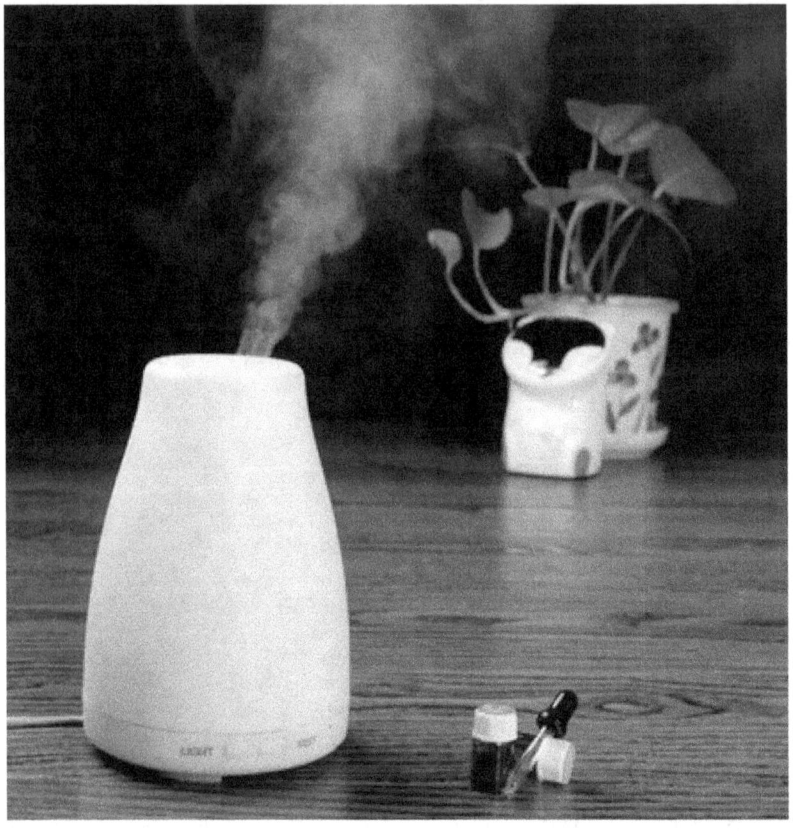

https : / / w w w . g o o g l e . c o m / s e a r c h ?
q=oil+diffuser&espv=2&biw=1366&bih=667&source=lnms&tbm=isch&sa=X&ved=0ahUKEwjC4IryqILNAhVS-
M1IKHVT9ClwQ_AUIBygC#imgrc=ANUjysqNITTJpM%3A

The most common method of using essential oils is diffusing. To do this, you purchase a diffuser, fill it with water (the amount of water varies with the diffuser you purchase), and add a few drops of oil.

If you know the specific symptom you want to treat, you put in the oil or blend of oils into the diffuser, plug it in, and let it fill the air with a delightful smelling mist. The aroma therapy treats the ailment, and makes your house smell incredible.

Topical use

Another prevalent method is applying the oil topically. When you do this, you still choose the oil you want based on the symptoms that are at hand. For example, you know that peppermint helps with stomach aches and lavender helps with restlessness, so if you are dealing with the stomach flu, a blend of these two oils will help a lot.

To apply topically, you are only going to use a few drops total, perhaps 2 drops of each oil.

Now, many oils are harsh applied directly to your skin, so you need to be careful with the oils you are using. The best way to prevent any skin irritation is to combine the oil with a carrier oil.

Carrier oils are mild oils that can be applied liberally to any part of your body, they are usually common oils such as coconut, sunflower, olive oil, or even vegetable oil if you are in a pinch.

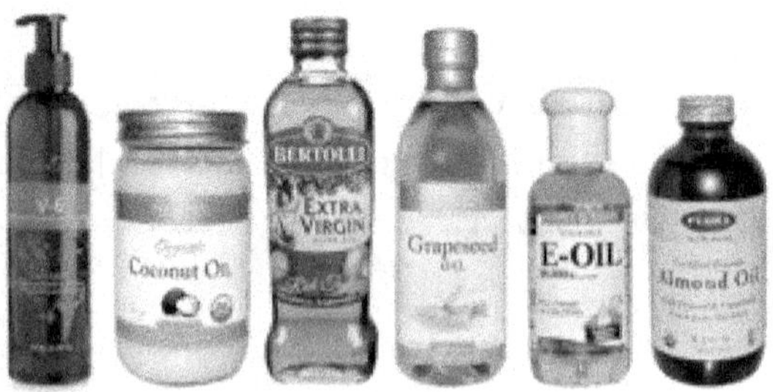

The best ratio I have found with the essential oil and the carrier oil is to combine a few drops of the essential oil with half a tablespoon of the carrier oil. Spread this on the part that is ailing (massage it into your forehead, onto your stomach, or any joint that is ailing. I find that it helps to warm the oil slightly before massaging it into your body.

Taking the Oil Internally

There is a lot of debate when it comes to ingesting essential oils. Many people advise against it because there can be harmful side effects, or you can overdose on the oils if you don't follow the dosages.

In my experience, I have never had an issue taking a couple drops of oil in my tea, but I am always careful of proper dosages. If you are going to use it in your tea, only use a couple of drops, no matter how big your cup of tea is. Only do this once a day.

Sure, there is the tendency to think that if 2 drops is good, then 4 must be better, but that is not the case. Essential oils are highly concentrated, which means the couple drops you are using in your tea is the equivalent to a lot of the fruit or other substance you are using.

Go mild, blend it into the tea you are drinking, and remember that less is more. If you feel sick, dizzy, or like something is off, discontinue ingesting the oils and simply use them topically or diffused into the air. There is evidence to support that you get the same benefits from using these oils topically or through aroma therapy as there is ingesting it.

At the end of the day, you get to decide what you want to do. It's your body, you get to decide. Don't be afraid to try out all three and decide which you want to do for yourself, and have fun with it!

My goal with this book is to give you the freedom you deserve to have with your health, and using essential oils is the best way to do that.

Chapter 6 – Good Mood Blends

In this book you are going to find all kinds of blends. You are going to find those that are fruity, those that embrace the wild side of the world, and those that grasp the musk and all of the natural scents that you simply must love.

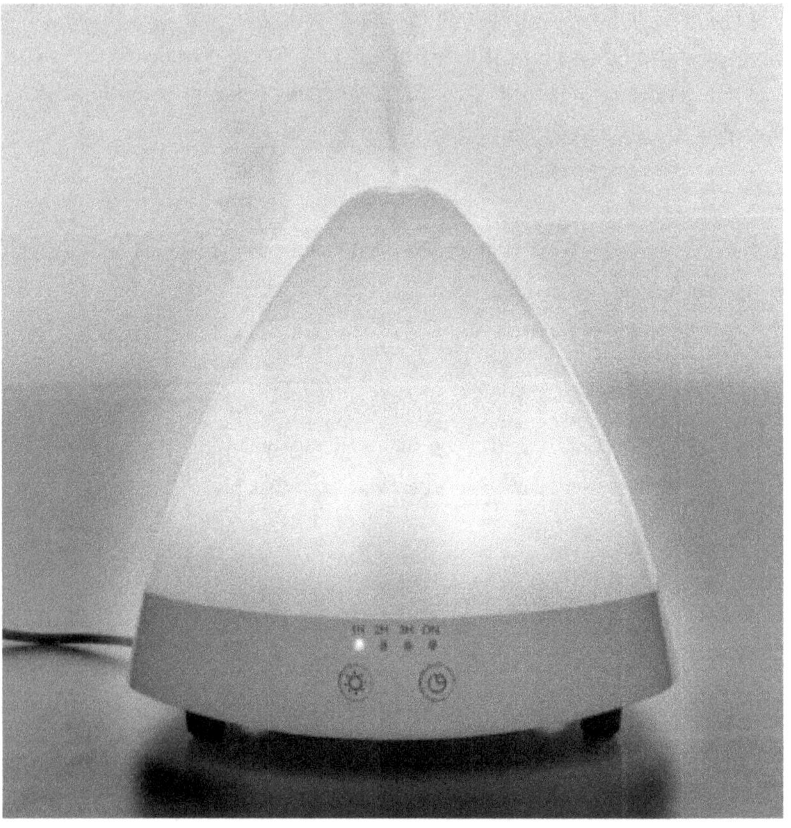

I want you to love each and every blend in this book, and by the time you work your way through all of the recipes, I want you to be in love with your diffuser as though it were one of your best friends in and of itself.

I don't ever want you to feel as though you are doing it wrong, or that you need something different to be happy with your oils. No matter what kind of diffuser you have, what kind of place you live in, or what your favorite scents are, this is the book that is for you.

Use these recipes as they are, use them for inspiration, or combine the two, but no matter what you do, have fun with it and fall in love with the finished product you craft.

The more happiness you feel as you blend, the more happiness is going to come out as you diffuse, and the better you are going to feel in your home. So grab that diffuser, and sit down with some tea, you are going to make happiness in a bottle as easy as one, two, three.

Sunshine Blend

5 drops lavender

5 drops hibiscus

5 drops lemongrass

Combine all the oils together in a glass jar, or directly into your diffuser. Fill your diffuser with water according to the size of your diffuser.

You can follow the recipe here as is, or you can feel free to modify to your own personal preference. Whatever you decide to do, have fun with it and love your blend!

Good Day Blend

5 drops rosewood

3 drops lemon

3 drops lemongrass

Combine all the oils together in a glass jar, or directly into your diffuser. Fill your diffuser with water according to the size of your diffuser.

You can follow the recipe here as is, or you can feel free to modify to your own personal preference. Whatever you decide to do, have fun with it and love your blend!

The Candyshop Blend

5 drops peppermint

3 drops lemon

3 drops rose

1 drop lavender

Combine all the oils together in a glass jar, or directly into your diffuser. Fill your diffuser with water according to the size of your diffuser.

You can follow the recipe here as is, or you can feel free to modify to your own personal preference. Whatever you decide to do, have fun with it and love your blend!

Money for my Honey

6 drops goldenseal

5 drops frankincense

3 drops rosewood

Combine all the oils together in a glass jar, or directly into your diffuser. Fill your diffuser with water according to the size of your diffuser.

You can follow the recipe here as is, or you can feel free to modify to your own personal preference. Whatever you decide to do, have fun with it and love your blend!

Fluffy Clouds

8 drops myrrh

5 drops goldenseal

3 drops orange

Combine all the oils together in a glass jar, or directly into your diffuser. Fill your diffuser with water according to the size of your diffuser.

You can follow the recipe here as is, or you can feel free to modify to your own personal preference. Whatever you decide to do, have fun with it and love your blend!

Peaceful Blend

8 drops agar

5 drops anise

5 drops rose

Combine all the oils together in a glass jar, or directly into your diffuser. Fill your diffuser with water according to the size of your diffuser.

You can follow the recipe here as is, or you can feel free to modify to your own personal preference. Whatever you decide to do, have fun with it and love your blend!

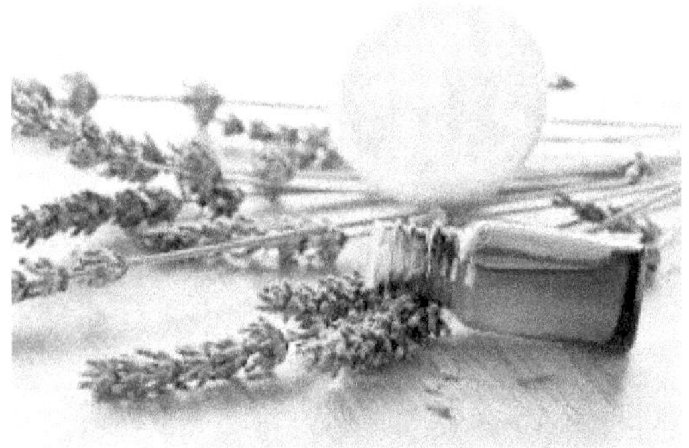

Thankfulness

8 drops bergamot

8 drops lime

5 drops lilac

Combine all the oils together in a glass jar, or directly into your diffuser. Fill your diffuser with water according to the size of your diffuser.

You can follow the recipe here as is, or you can feel free to modify to your own personal preference. Whatever you decide to do, have fun with it and love your blend!

Smiles and Laughter

8 drops anise

8 drops geranium

5 drops black pepper

Combine all the oils together in a glass jar, or directly into your diffuser. Fill your diffuser with water according to the size of your diffuser.

You can follow the recipe here as is, or you can feel free to modify to your own personal preference. Whatever you decide to do, have fun with it and love your blend!

Chapter 7 – All The Spice And Twice As Nice

When you think of happiness and the scents that go along with the feeling, you may start to think of such things as parties, beaches, fairs, the ocean, and things along those lines.

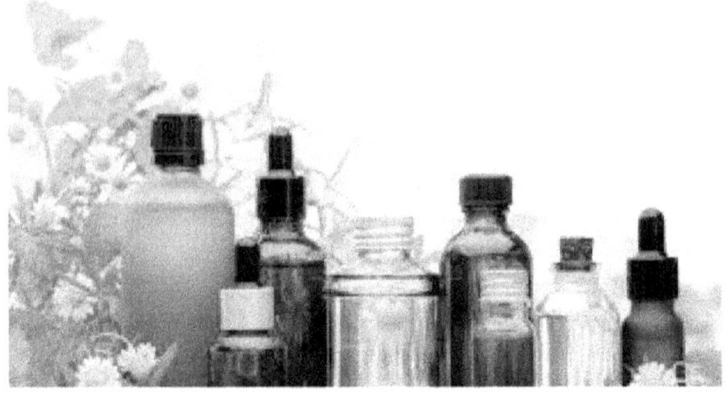

https://www.google.com/search?q=diffuser&espv=2&biw=1366&bih=667&site=webhp&source=lnms&tbm=isch&sa=X&ved=0ahUKEwi2ybOGjvLNAh-UHLmMKHbomCEMQ_AUIBygC#imgrc=Rptq34BLaMbFyM%3A

And there is nothing at all wrong with that, those are all incredible places to go and fun things to do, and they are more often than not the things most associate with good feelings, but I want to challenge you to take a step out of the norm.

Don't think that you have to be at the beach to have fun, but embrace the world around you. Think of the dark, musky scents that the earth brings. Go out into your garden, into the fields, and into anywhere you can think of where you can breathe in the rustic smell of trees, dust, and soil.

You are going to find a whole new level of happiness you never thought of before, and you will want to capture that scent for your own home.

With these blends, you are going to get a glimpse of that musk anywhere in your house that you want, and anytime you want, you can escape to that happy place where you embrace nature for all that it is.

And you will never want to walk away.

Arabian Nights

8 drops sandalwood

5 drops myrrh

5 drops patchouli

Combine all the oils together in a glass jar, or directly into your diffuser. Fill your diffuser with water according to the size of your diffuser.

You can follow the recipe here as is, or you can feel free to modify to your own personal preference. Whatever you decide to do, have fun with it and love your blend!

Spice Girl Life Blend

10 drops cinnamon

5 drops ginger

5 drops sandalwood

Combine all the oils together in a glass jar, or directly into your diffuser. Fill your diffuser with water according to the size of your diffuser.

You can follow the recipe here as is, or you can feel free to modify to your own personal preference. Whatever you decide to do, have fun with it and love your blend!

Magic Musky Moonlight

8 drops cardamom

7 drops cedar

7 drops chamomile

Combine all the oils together in a glass jar, or directly into your diffuser. Fill your diffuser with water according to the size of your diffuser.

You can follow the recipe here as is, or you can feel free to modify to your own personal preference. Whatever you decide to do, have fun with it and love your blend!

The Dessert Spice Blend

6 drops clary sage

8 drops sandalwood

5 drops calamus

Combine all the oils together in a glass jar, or directly into your diffuser. Fill your diffuser with water according to the size of your diffuser.

You can follow the recipe here as is, or you can feel free to modify to your own personal preference. Whatever you decide to do, have fun with it and love your blend!

Spice Cake Surprise

6 drops cinnamon

6 drops clove oil

5 drops garlic oil

5 drops ginger

Combine all the oils together in a glass jar, or directly into your diffuser. Fill your diffuser with water according to the size of your diffuser.

You can follow the recipe here as is, or you can feel free to modify to your own personal preference. Whatever you decide to do, have fun with it and love your blend!

The Wood Fairies

5 drops rosewood

5 drops cedar wood

8 drops sandalwood

5 drops pine

Combine all the oils together in a glass jar, or directly into your diffuser. Fill your diffuser with water according to the size of your diffuser.

You can follow the recipe here as is, or you can feel free to modify to your own personal preference. Whatever you decide to do, have fun with it and love your blend!

Magic Music

6 drops jasmine

5 drops hyssop

5 drops neem oil

Combine all the oils together in a glass jar, or directly into your diffuser. Fill your diffuser with water according to the size of your diffuser.

You can follow the recipe here as is, or you can feel free to modify to your own personal preference. Whatever you decide to do, have fun with it and love your blend!

The Richness of the Earth

7 drops patchouli

5 drops red cedar

4 drops lemongrass

2 drops rosehip

Combine all the oils together in a glass jar, or directly into your diffuser. Fill your diffuser with water according to the size of your diffuser.

You can follow the recipe here as is, or you can feel free to modify to your own personal preference. Whatever you decide to do, have fun with it and love your blend!

Chapter 8 – Beautiful Day Blends

Few things in life are able to compare to the beauty of a wonderful day. It doesn't need to be anything in particular that makes the day wonderful, but perhaps you are happy to be alive, and you let your happiness overflow into the world around you.

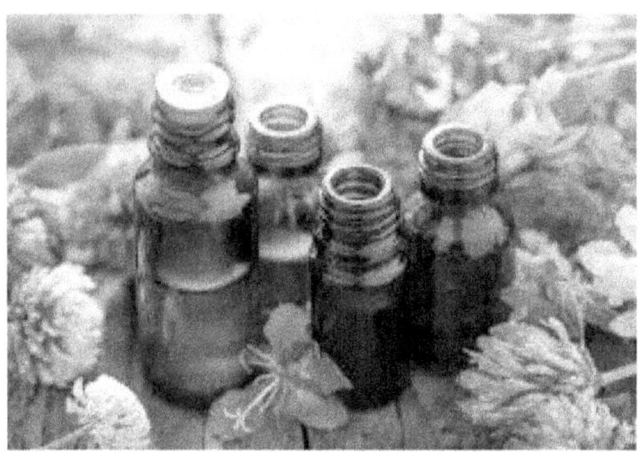

https://www.google.com/search?q=diffuser&espv=2&biw=1366&bih=667&site=webhp&source=lnms&tbm=isch&sa=X&ved=0ahUKEwi2ybOGjvLNAh-UHLmMKHbomCEMQ_AUIBygC#imgrc=Rptq34BLaMbFyM%3A

You know that good vibes and happiness are the best things to spread to the world, so why not start with your own home and create a place where good vibes and excellent scents go hand in hand?

You are going to feel as though you escaped to a wonderful fairy garden when you walk into any room of your house, breathing in the deep, crisp scent of any one of these oil blends.

Have fun and let your worries melt away. There is nothing that can compare with these.

Pixels and Pixies

3 drops hibiscus

4 drops rosewood

3 drops basil

3 drops sage

Combine all the oils together in a glass jar, or directly into your diffuser. Fill your diffuser with water according to the size of your diffuser.

You can follow the recipe here as is, or you can feel free to modify to your own personal preference. Whatever you decide to do, have fun with it and love your blend!

A Walk Around The Block

4 drops cedar

4 drops cedarwood

5 drops clary sage

5 drops sage

Combine all the oils together in a glass jar, or directly into your diffuser. Fill your diffuser with water according to the size of your diffuser.

You can follow the recipe here as is, or you can feel free to modify to your own personal preference. Whatever you decide to do, have fun with it and love your blend!

Bees and Butterflies

6 drops spruce

6 drops tangerine

6 drops pine

Combine all the oils together in a glass jar, or directly into your diffuser. Fill your diffuser with water according to the size of your diffuser.

You can follow the recipe here as is, or you can feel free to modify to your own personal preference. Whatever you decide to do, have fun with it and love your blend!

The Gently Blowing Breeze

8 drops patchouli

8 drops lemongrass

4 drops tea tree

5 drops tarragon

Combine all the oils together in a glass jar, or directly into your diffuser. Fill your diffuser with water according to the size of your diffuser.

You can follow the recipe here as is, or you can feel free to modify to your own personal preference. Whatever you decide to do, have fun with it and love your blend!

Fresh Linen on the Line

5 drops peppermint

5 drops eucalyptus

6 drops tangerine

5 drops spearmint

Combine all the oils together in a glass jar, or directly into your diffuser. Fill your diffuser with water according to the size of your diffuser.

You can follow the recipe here as is, or you can feel free to modify to your own personal preference. Whatever you decide to do, have fun with it and love your blend!

Raindrops on the Roses

10 drops eucalyptus

8 drops rosewood

8 drops rose

5 drops sage

Combine all the oils together in a glass jar, or directly into your diffuser. Fill your diffuser with water according to the size of your diffuser.

You can follow the recipe here as is, or you can feel free to modify to your own personal preference. Whatever you decide to do, have fun with it and love your blend!

The Flower Garden

10 drops lavender

10 drops rose

6 drops hibiscus

6 drops lilac

5 drops lemon

5 drops tangerine

Combine all the oils together in a glass jar, or directly into your diffuser. Fill your diffuser with water according to the size of your diffuser.

You can follow the recipe here as is, or you can feel free to modify to your own personal preference. Whatever you decide to do, have fun with it and love your blend!

Umbrella on my Shoulders

10 drops orange

5 drops blood orange

5 drops lime oil

4 drops eucalyptus

Combine all the oils together in a glass jar, or directly into your diffuser. Fill your diffuser with water according to the size of your diffuser.

You can follow the recipe here as is, or you can feel free to modify to your own personal preference. Whatever you decide to do, have fun with it and love your blend!

Chapter 9 – The Best Blends For A Helpful Kick

There's nothing better than a blend that is able to bring life to your house, and fill your house with all kinds of good things in addition to the good vibes you get when you breathe deeply.

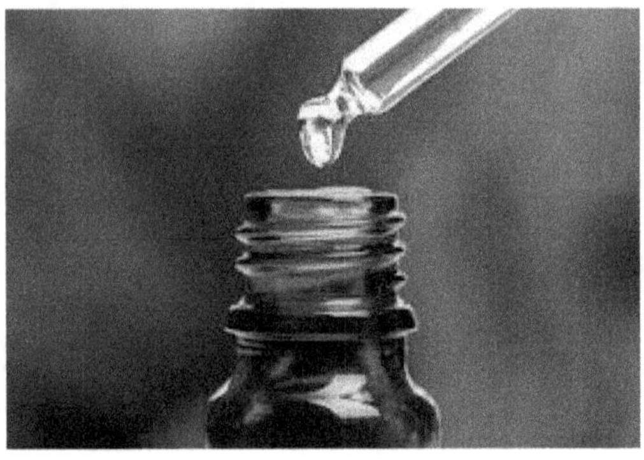

https://www.google.com/search?q=diffuser&espv=2&biw=1366&bih=667&site=webhp&source=lnms&tbm=isch&sa=X&ved=0ahUKEwi2ybOGjvLNAh-UHLmMKHbomCEMQ_AUIBygC#imgrc=Rptq34BLaMbFyM%3A

I crafted a blend of the finest scents to bring smiles to your face, but I have also chosen the best oils for headaches, joint pain, and tension. I wanted to fill your home with not only the great, fresh scents that only these oils can bring, but also the peach and relaxation that they possess as well.

When you add these oils to your diffuser, you are combining just what you need to make your home not only delicious and welcoming to all who enter, but you are creating an oasis from the world. A place where you can feel relaxed, pain free, and able to enjoy yourself without any form of tension whatsoever.

So if you want to embrace your own version of a nirvana island, grab your diffuser and these oils, plus a few more of your own if you want to bring in that personal touch.

Toss them into the mix, close your eyes, and sit back to enjoy all of the great benefits of these oils.

The Headache Buster

10 drops peppermint

10 drops eucalyptus

5 drops wintergreen

5 drops spearmint

Combine all the oils together in a glass jar, or directly into your diffuser. Fill your diffuser with water according to the size of your diffuser.

You can follow the recipe here as is, or you can feel free to modify to your own personal preference. Whatever you decide to do, have fun with it and love your blend!

The Immunity Booster

5 drops frankincense

4 drops lemon

4 drops eucalyptus

5 drops garlic

10 drops tea tree

Combine all the oils together in a glass jar, or directly into your diffuser. Fill your diffuser with water according to the size of your diffuser.

You can follow the recipe here as is, or you can feel free to modify to your own personal preference. Whatever you decide to do, have fun with it and love your blend!

The Calming Blend

10 drops vetiver

5 drops lavender

5 drops peppermint

2 drops spearmint

Combine all the oils together in a glass jar, or directly into your diffuser. Fill your diffuser with water according to the size of your diffuser.

You can follow the recipe here as is, or you can feel free to modify to your own personal preference. Whatever you decide to do, have fun with it and love your blend!

The Life of the Party

10 drops lemongrass

4 drops lemon

4 drops tangerine

5 drops sweet orange

5 drops orange

Combine all the oils together in a glass jar, or directly into your diffuser. Fill your diffuser with water according to the size of your diffuser.

You can follow the recipe here as is, or you can feel free to modify to your own personal preference. Whatever you decide to do, have fun with it and love your blend!

The Fixer Fizzer

8 drops tea tree

8 drops peppermint

4 drops myrrh

4 drops cardamom

Combine all the oils together in a glass jar, or directly into your diffuser. Fill your diffuser with water according to the size of your diffuser.

You can follow the recipe here as is, or you can feel free to modify to your own personal preference. Whatever you decide to do, have fun with it and love your blend!

The All In One Blend

5 drops goldenseal

10 drops grapefruit

4 drops ginger

4 drops cinnamon

Combine all the oils together in a glass jar, or directly into your diffuser. Fill your diffuser with water according to the size of your diffuser.

You can follow the recipe here as is, or you can feel free to modify to your own personal preference. Whatever you decide to do, have fun with it and love your blend!

Aches and Pains Melt Away Blend

11 drops lavender

11 drops spruce

5 drops cedar wood

5 drops grapefruit

Combine all the oils together in a glass jar, or directly into your diffuser. Fill your diffuser with water according to the size of your diffuser.

You can follow the recipe here as is, or you can feel free to modify to your own personal preference. Whatever you decide to do, have fun with it and love your blend!

The Bedroom Blend

10 drops peppermint

5 drops cinnamon

5 drops wintergreen

5 drops spruce

Combine all the oils together in a glass jar, or directly into your diffuser. Fill your diffuser with water according to the size of your diffuser.

You can follow the recipe here as is, or you can feel free to modify to your own personal preference. Whatever you decide to do, have fun with it and love your blend!

Chapter 10 – Unique Blends For The Uniquely You

The best way to describe any of the blends in this chapter is with the word unique. There is something simply delightful but entirely one of a kind about each of the blends, and I highly encourage you to add your little touch of personality to any or all of them.

Have fun with it, use your imagination, and use as little or as much of any of the oils as you wish. If you think that there's another little something that would bring out the right note, toss it into the mix!

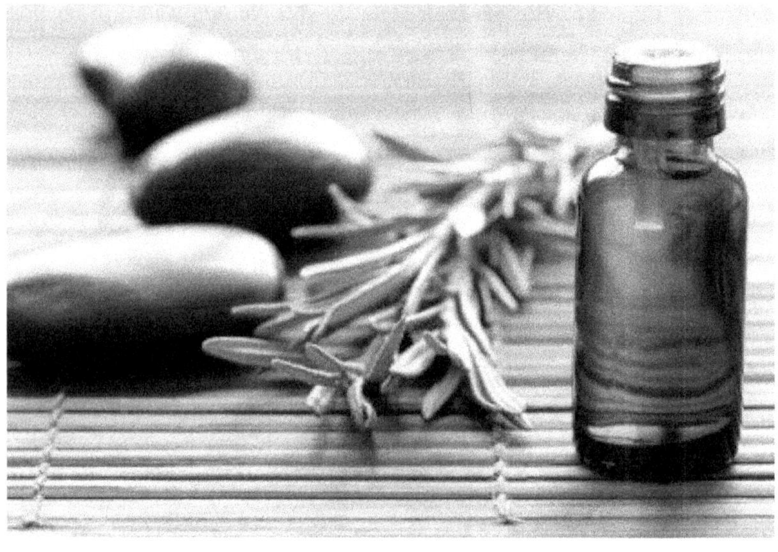

You can't go wrong with it, and if you are in love, then the blend is the perfect blend for you.

Just What You Needed Blend

8 drops cinnamon

7 drops orange

5 drops patchouli

3 drops spruce

Combine all the oils together in a glass jar, or directly into your diffuser. Fill your diffuser with water according to the size of your diffuser.

You can follow the recipe here as is, or you can feel free to modify to your own personal preference. Whatever you decide to do, have fun with it and love your blend!

Yours Truly Blend

10 drops rose

8 drops lavender

3 drops spearmint

3 drops grapefruit

3 drops tea tree oil

Combine all the oils together in a glass jar, or directly into your diffuser. Fill your diffuser with water according to the size of your diffuser.

You can follow the recipe here as is, or you can feel free to modify to your own personal preference. Whatever you decide to do, have fun with it and love your blend!

Anything and Everything

8 drops frankincense

4 drops spikenard

4 drops patchouli

4 drops vetiver

3 drops spruce

Combine all the oils together in a glass jar, or directly into your diffuser. Fill your diffuser with water according to the size of your diffuser.

You can follow the recipe here as is, or you can feel free to modify to your own personal preference. Whatever you decide to do, have fun with it and love your blend!

Everything You Wanted Blend

9 drops ylang ylang

5 drops tangerine

5 drops wintergreen

4 drops cedar wood

Combine all the oils together in a glass jar, or directly into your diffuser. Fill your diffuser with water according to the size of your diffuser.

You can follow the recipe here as is, or you can feel free to modify to your own personal preference. Whatever you decide to do, have fun with it and love your blend!

You and Me is Three Blend

4 drops tea tree

8 drops grapefruit

8 drops cinnamon

Combine all the oils together in a glass jar, or directly into your diffuser. Fill your diffuser with water according to the size of your diffuser.

You can follow the recipe here as is, or you can feel free to modify to your own personal preference. Whatever you decide to do, have fun with it and love your blend!

Your Dream Come True Blend

8 drops lavender

9 drops spruce

4 drops ylang ylang

3 drops tea tree

Combine all the oils together in a glass jar, or directly into your diffuser. Fill your diffuser with water according to the size of your diffuser.

You can follow the recipe here as is, or you can feel free to modify to your own personal preference. Whatever you decide to do, have fun with it and love your blend!

The Super Spoiler Blend

12 drops ylang ylang

6 drops vetiver

4 drops myrrh

4 drops patchouli

Combine all the oils together in a glass jar, or directly into your diffuser. Fill your diffuser with water according to the size of your diffuser.

You can follow the recipe here as is, or you can feel free to modify to your own personal preference. Whatever you decide to do, have fun with it and love your blend!

Indulgence in Love Blend

7 drops cinnamon

4 drops rose

4 drops tangerine

2 drops spearmint

2 drops tea tree oil

Combine all the oils together in a glass jar, or directly into your diffuser. Fill your diffuser with water according to the size of your diffuser.

You can follow the recipe here as is, or you can feel free to modify to your own personal preference. Whatever you decide to do, have fun with it and love your blend!

Chapter 10. Summer & Spring Essential Oil Diffuser Recipes

Why to opt for natural essential oil diffusers?

The herbs which are used for the extraction of essential oils are very much beneficial and are being in use for centuries. The oils are mostly extracted from the
herbs and plants and are used for multiple purposes. The essential oils are extracted from various origins like orange peel, lemon peel, almond, lavender, eucalyptus etc. There is a much wider exposure of humans to these essential oils
which are chemical free. The main benefit of using these essential oils for the
treatment of anything is that these oils are completely deprived of any harmful or
side effect thus you can use them in any way and for getting anything cured.

Exceptional properties

Not only this, but many of the essential oils have also got the property of having
extra ordinary fragrance, so these oils can also be used as a fragrance and a very
good example of such a fragrance is the rose essential oil, which is not only used
for the tremens of various skin problems but also used as a fragrance and as an
essential part of many concentrated perfumes.

Thus we can say that the essential oils have got immense importance which cannot be denied in any case and if you want to get all the bandits out of these oils
you must follow all the steps and techniques of using the essential oils for treatment of any problem.

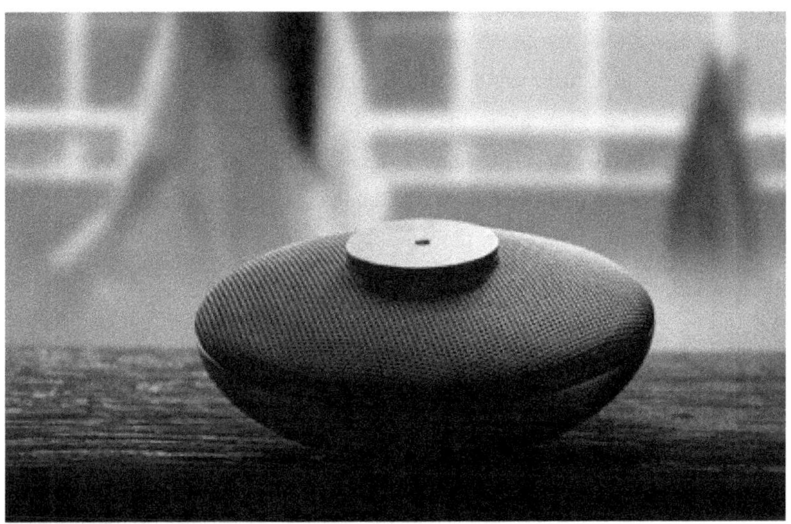

As far as the extent of choosing the right oils are concerned for making right fragrance, it is basically up to you that what kind of fragrance do you like and what are those ingredients which you want to be added as an essential component of deodorant you are making. Sometimes, you cannot become able to decide what to do with the ingredients you have. But do not worry at all as I have given the exact and perfect combination of different oils so that different types of fragrances can be made out of them.

The idea behind choosing the diffusers which I will be giving you in the coming chapters lies in the fact that I was thinking about different occasions where some kind of festivity or joy will be or different types of mood which I may have depending upon the environment in which I am present. So, you must be having the same thinking for sure as for different occasions you will be having different moods as well.

The diffusers which are manufactured synthetically can be composed of some harmful chemicals which can harm your skin and which should not be taken in to your consideration when you are looking for some diffuser in any local store near you. So, you are just in a need of having some organic essential oils so that you can use them without facing any problem.

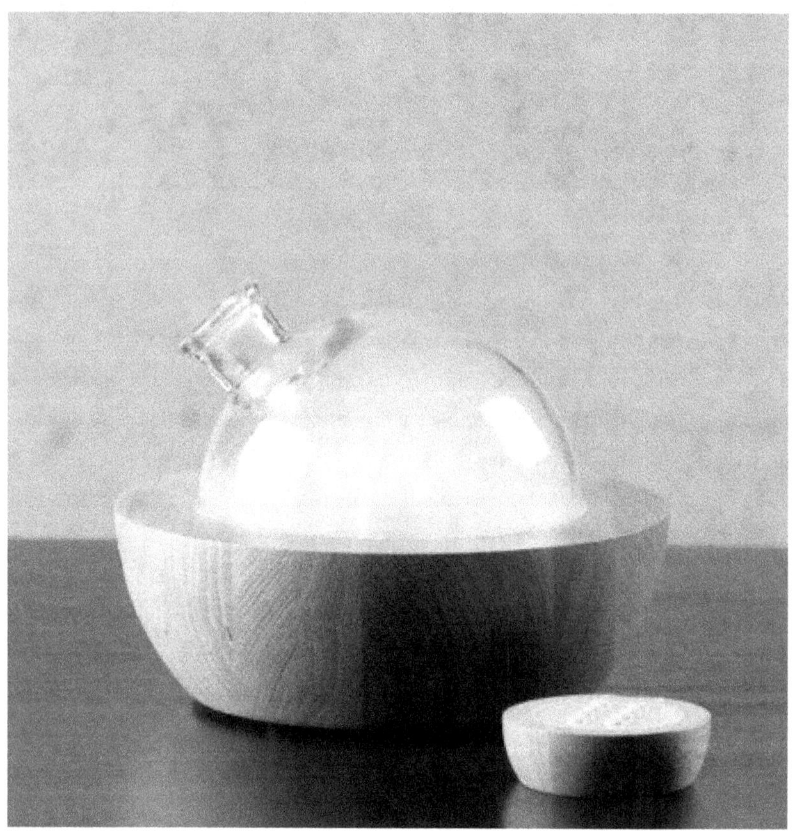

One important aspect of homemade diffuser is that, you can have their fragrance with you for quite a longer period of time, sometimes for all day, unlike that of synthetic diffusers who may disappear just after some time.

It is true that all of us having a desire of smelling something good which is good in fragrance and which is liked by everyone. If you get to have your own diffuser of your own then it will really be that thing full of fun for you when you will use it in routine at so many occasions and for so many reasons. This signature secret will make you able to have some unique value of yours as compared to the people who are around you as it is that smell that is exclusively being used by you and not by anyone else.

At this stage, you should not forget this in any case that when you are going to make your own diffuser with the help of organic ingredients, you should be patient enough to look for the right things to do. Do not do anything which can take you towards hurry and be there to exhibit patience as some diffuser require some days to get in to that consistency which you are desiring to have with you.

20 essential oil diffuser recipes

Recipe no. 1

Ingredients:

- Jojoba oil three drops

- Almond oil four drops

- Jasmine essential oil four drops

Method:

- Take all the oils that have been mentioned in the detailed list of ingredients and their quantity above.

- Beware that you are taking the right quantity just according to what have been mentioned in the ingredients above.

- Leave the bottle for about four days in a dry place or you can also place it in the sun for four to four hours daily so that all the oils get mixed with each other with a high level of consistency.

- Then keep the bottle at a place with the lowest level of humidity.

Recipe no. 2

Ingredients:

- Honey three drops

- Jojoba oil three drops

- Carrot oil four drops

- Jasmine essential oil four drops

- Lemon oil three drops

Method:

- Take all the oils that have been mentioned in the detailed list of ingredients and their quantity above.

- Take a small bottle or container and add all the above-mentioned ingredients.

- Close the lid of the bottle and mix the oils very well.

- Leave the bottle for about four to three days so that all the oils get mixed with each other with a high level of consistency.

- Then keep the bottle in cool and dry place.

- Place the diffuser cap at the top of the bottle.

- Press the button to have its fumes out whenever you need.

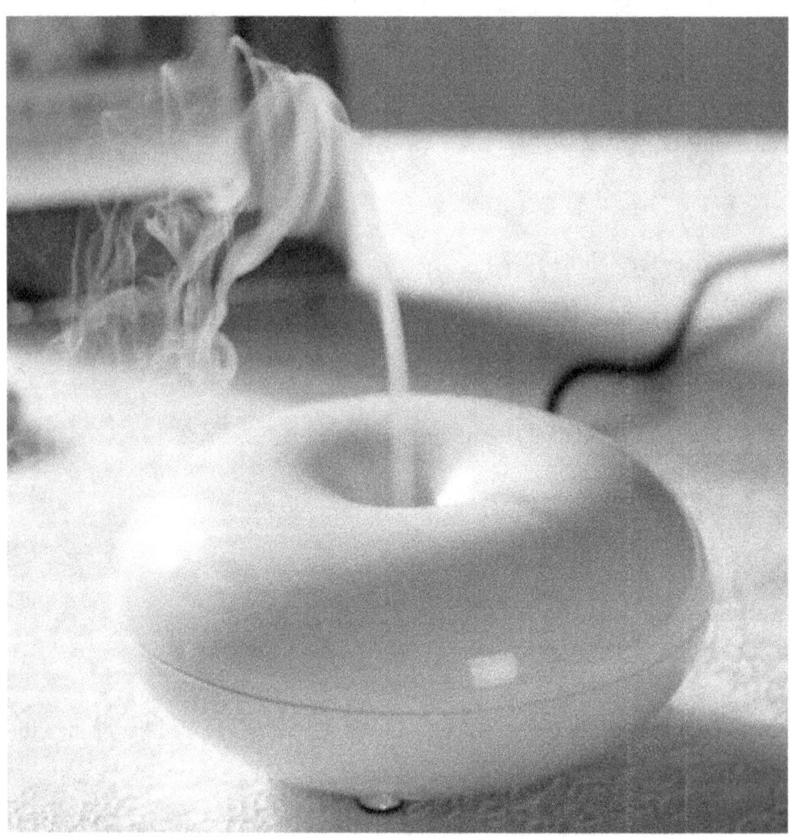

Recipe no. 3

Ingredients:

- Jojoba oil three drops

- Almond oil four drops

- Rose essential oil four drops

- Lemon oil four drops

Method:

- Take all the oils that have been mentioned in the detailed list of ingredients and their quantity above.

- Make the lid of the bottle closed and mix the oils well so that they can become smooth in consistency.

- Leave the bottle for about one day or 24 hours in a dry place or you can also place it in the sun for four to four hours daily so that all the oils get mixed with each other with a high level of consistency.

- Then keep the bottle at a place with the lowest level of humidity.

- Place the diffuser cap at the top of the bottle.

- Press the button to have its fumes out whenever you need.

Recipe no. 4

Ingredients:

- Lemon oil three drops

- Almond oil three drops

- Jojoba oil five drops

- Jasmine essential oil four drops

Method:

- Take all the oils that have been mentioned in the detailed list of ingredients and their quantity above.

- Take a small bottle or container and add all the ingredients that have been mentioned in the above-mentioned list for your convenience.

- Close the bottle's lid tightly so that no air can enter inside and mix all the mixtures well so that you can get the desired consistency out of it without any ambiguity on your way.

- Leave the bottle for about three to five days so that all the oils get mixed with each other with a high level of consistency.

- Place the diffuser cap at the top of the bottle.

- Press the button to have its fumes out whenever you need.

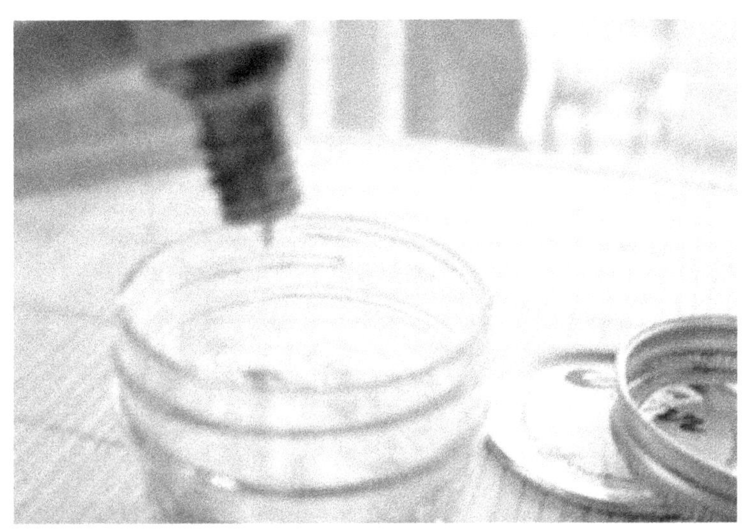

Recipe no. 5

Ingredients:

- Jojoba oil three drops

- Jasmine essential oil three drops

- Lemon oil four drops

- Almond oil four drops

Method:

- Take all the oils that have been mentioned in the detailed list of ingredients and their quantity above.

- Take a small bottle or container and add all the ingredients that have been mentioned in the above-mentioned list for your convenience.

- Make the lid of the bottle closed and mix the oils well so that they can become smooth in consistency.

- Now you should keep the bottle in dry place for about two to three days, so that all the ingredients get consistent.

- Place the diffuser cap at the top of the bottle.

- Press the button to have its fumes out whenever you need.

Recipe no. 6

Ingredients:

- Grapefruit oil three drops

- Jasmine essential oil four drops

- Sweet almond oil three drops

- Rose essential oil four drops

Method:

- Take all the oils that have been mentioned in the detailed list of ingredients and their quantity above.

- Beware that you are taking the right quantity just according to what have been mentioned in the ingredients above.

- Take a small bottle or container and add all the ingredients that have been mentioned in the above-mentioned list for your convenience.

- Leave the bottle for about four days in a dry place or you can also place it in the sun for four to four hours daily so that all the oils get mixed with each other with a high level of consistency.

- Place the diffuser cap at the top of the bottle.

- Press the button to have its fumes out whenever you need.

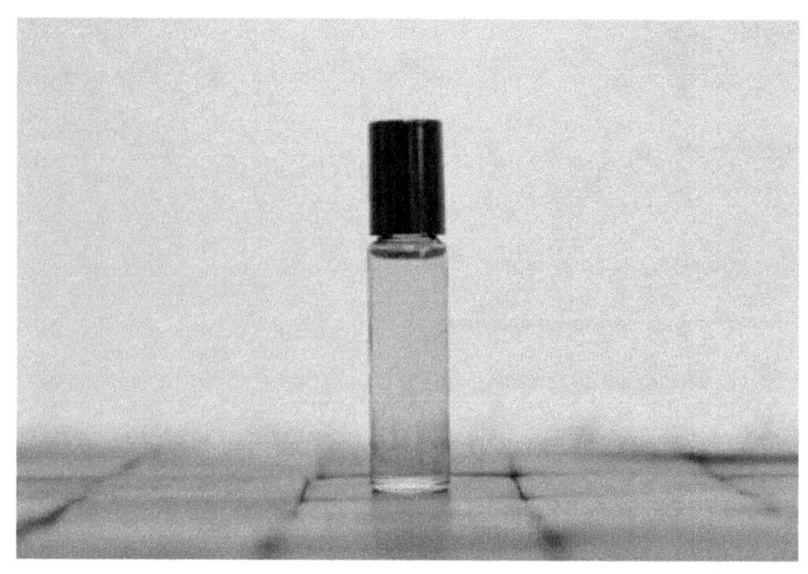

Recipe no. 7

Ingredients:

- Almond oil three drops
- Almond oil three drops
- Jasmine oil four drops
- Jasmine essential oil four drops

Method:

- Take all the oils that have been mentioned in the detailed list of ingredients.
- Beware that you are taking the right quantity as it is mentioned above.
- Take a small bottle or container and add all the ingredients that have been mentioned in the above-mentioned list for your convenience.
- Place the diffuser cap at the top of the bottle.
- Press the button to have its fumes out, whenever you need.

Recipe no. 8

Ingredients:

- Nutmeg oil three drops

- Rosemary oil four drops

- Jasmine essential oil four drops

- Almond oil four drops

- Black cumin oil four drops

Method:

- Take all the oils that have been above.

- Close the bottle's lid tightly so that no air can enter inside and mix all the mixtures well so that you can get the desired consistency out of it without any ambiguity on your way.

- Now you should keep the bottle in dry place for about two to three days, so that all the ingredients get consistent.

- Then keep the bottle in cool place.

- Place the diffuser cap at the top of the bottle.

- Press the button to have its fumes out whenever you need.

- Apply it to neck, back of year and wrist to get elegant fragrance.

Recipe no. 9

Ingredients:

- Lavender oil four drops

- Almond oil three drops

- Jojoba oil four drops

- Lemon oil three drops

Method:

- Take all the ingredients mentioned above in a small bottle with a cap.

- Beware that you are taking the right quantity just according to what have been mentioned in the ingredients above.

- Take a small bottle or container and add all the ingredients that have been mentioned in the above-mentioned list for your convenience.

- Now you should keep the bottle in dry place for about two to three days, so that all the ingredients get consistent.

- Place the diffuser cap at the top of the bottle.

- Press the button to have its fumes out whenever you need.

- Apply it to neck, back of year and wrist to get elegant fragrance.

Recipe no. 10

Ingredients:

- Almond oil three drops

- Cilantro oil four drops

- Jasmine essential oil 2 drops

Method:

- Take all the ingredients mentioned above in a small bottle with a cap.

- Beware that you are taking the right quantity as it is mentioned above.

- Close the bottle's lid tightly so that no air can enter inside and mix all the mixtures well.

- Place the diffuser cap at the top of the bottle.

- Press the button to have its fumes out whenever you need.

- Apply the body spray at the back of the ear, in front of neck, on the chest or at any place of your body where you are having the desire to apply it.

Recipe no. 11

Ingredients:

- Almond oil 3 teaspoon
- Lemon juice 3 drops
- Jasmine essential oil 3 drops
- Lemon oil 3 drops

Method:

- Take a small container and add all the ingredients that have been mentioned above.
- Close the cap of the container and mix the oils well.
- Leave the container for about 3 days so that the body spray can be enriched.
- Place the diffuser cap at the top of the bottle.
- Press the button to have its fumes out whenever you need.
- Apply the body spray at the back of the ear, in front of neck, or at any place of your body where you want.

Recipe no. 12

Ingredients:

- Rosemary oil 3 drops

- Almond oil 3 drops

- Raspberry essential oil 3 drops

- Jasmine essential oil 9 drops

Method:

- Take a small container and add all the ingredients that have been mentioned above.

- Make the cap of the bottle closed and mix the oils well so that they can become smooth in consistency.

- Leave the bottle for about 5 days in a dry place or you can also place it in the sun for 3 to 3 hours daily so that the body spray can be enriched.

- Then keep the bottle at a place with the lowest level of humidity.

- Place the diffuser cap at the top of the bottle.

- Press the button to have its fumes out whenever you need.

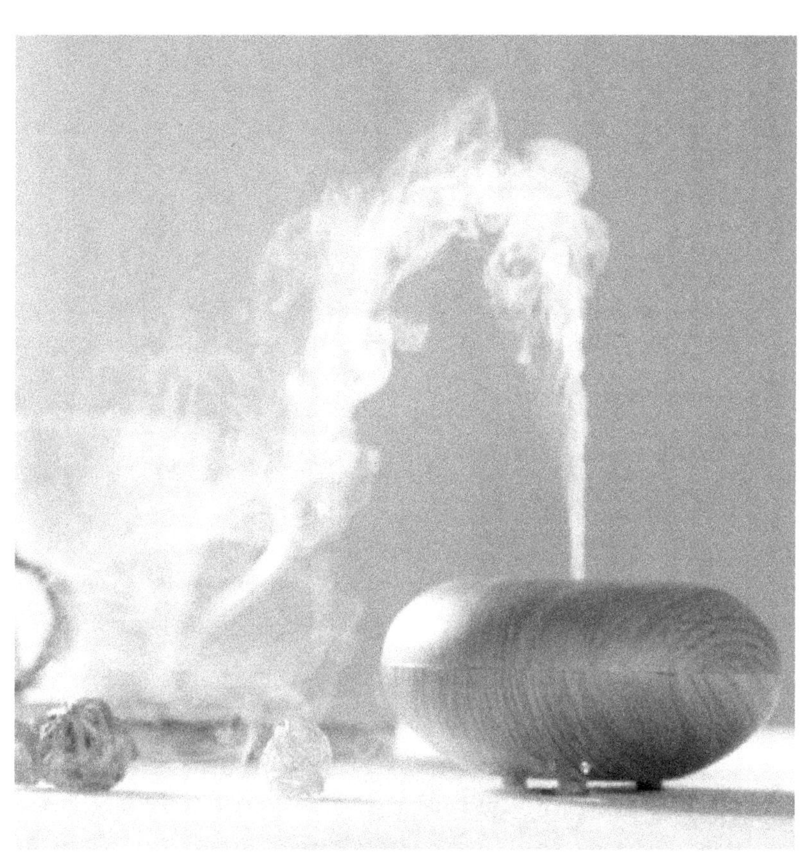

Recipe no. 13

Ingredients:

- Cumin oil 3 drops

- Ginger oil 3 drops

- Grapefruit oil 3 drops

- Jasmine essential oil 3 drops

- Raspberry essential oil 3 drops

Method:

- Take a small container and add all the ingredients that have been mentioned above.

- Close the bottle's cap tightly so that no air can enter inside and mix all the mixtures well so that you can get the desired consistency out of it without any ambiguity on your way.

- Leave the bottle for about 3 days so that the body spray can be enriched.

- Then keep the bottle in cool and dry place.

- Place the diffuser cap at the top of the bottle.

- Press the button to have its fumes out whenever you need.

Recipe no. 14

Ingredients:

- Rosemary oil 3 drops
- Almond oil 3 drops
- Raspberry essential oil 3 drops
- Jasmine essential oil 3 drops

Method:

- Take all the oils that have been mentioned in the detailed list of ingredients and their quantity above.
- Beware that you are taking the right quantity as it is mentioned above.
- Close the bottle's cap tightly so that no air can enter inside.
- Mix all the mixtures well so that you can get the desired consistency out of it.
- Then keep the bottle in cool and dry place.
- Place the diffuser cap at the top of the bottle.
- Press the button to have its fumes out whenever you need.

Recipe no. 15

Ingredients:

- Almond oil 3 drops

- Cilantro oil 3 drops

- Jasmine essential oil 3 drops

- Raspberry essential oil 3 drops

- Cumin oil 3 drops

Method:

- Take a small bottle or container and add all the ingredients that have been mentioned in the above-mentioned list for your convenience.

- Make the cap of the bottle closed and mix the oils well so that they can become smooth in consistency.

- Leave the bottle for about 3 days in a dry place or you can also place it in the sun for 3 to 3 hours daily so that the body spray can be enriched.

- Then keep the bottle at a place with the lowest level of humidity. Place the diffuser cap at the top of the bottle.

- Press the button to have its fumes out whenever you need.

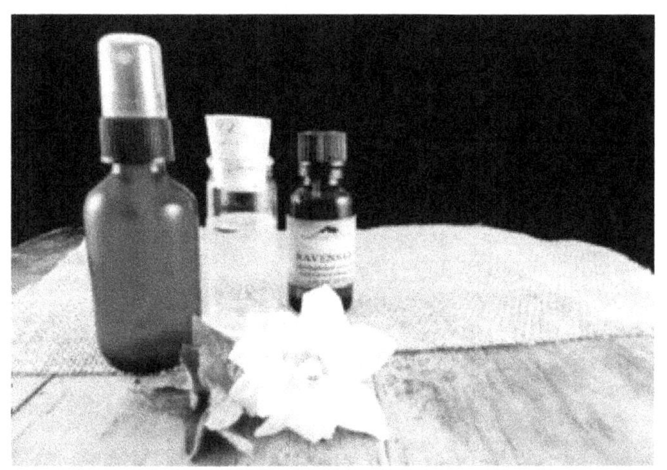

Recipe no. 16

Ingredients:

- Rose essential oil 3 drops

- Jasmine essential oil 3 drops

- Cumin oil 3 drops

- Lemon oil 3 drops

- Savory oil 3 drops

Method:

- Take a small bottle or container and add all the ingredients that have been mentioned in the above-mentioned list for your convenience.

- Close the bottle's cap tightly so that no air can enter inside and mix all the mixtures well so that you can get the desired consistency out of it without any ambiguity on your way.

- Then keep the bottle in cool and dry place.

- Place the diffuser cap at the top of the bottle.

- Press the button to have its fumes out whenever you need.

Recipe no. 17

Ingredients:

- Almond essential oil 3 teaspoon

- Turmeric oil 3 drops

- Clementine oil 3 drops

- Clove bud oil 3 drops

Method:

- Take a small bottle or container and add all the ingredients that have been mentioned in the above-mentioned list for your convenience.

- Make the cap of the bottle closed and mix the oils well so that they can become smooth in consistency.

- Leave the bottle for about 3 days in a dry place or you can also place it in the sun for 3 to 3 hours daily so that the body spray can be enriched.

- Then keep the bottle at a place with the lowest level of humidity.

- Place the diffuser cap at the top of the bottle.

- Press the button to have its fumes out whenever you need.

Recipe no. 18

Ingredients:

- Rose essential oil 3 drops

- Rosemary essential oil 3 teaspoon

- Jasmine essential oil 3 teaspoon

- Apple cider vinegar half cup

Method:

- Take a small bottle or container and add all the ingredients that have been mentioned in the above-mentioned list for your convenience.

- Close the bottle's cap tightly so that no air can enter inside and mix all the mixtures well so that you can get the desired consistency out of it without any ambiguity on your way.

- Place the diffuser cap at the top of the bottle.

- Press the button to have its fumes out whenever you need.

Recipe no. 19

Ingredients:

- Coconut oil 3 teaspoon
- Rosemary essential oil 3 teaspoon
- Lemongrass oil 3 teaspoon
- Cumin oil 3 drops
- Vanilla oil 3 drops
- Sage oil 3 drops

Method:

- Take all the oils and ingredients.
- Take a small bottle or container and add all the ingredients that have been mentioned in the above-mentioned list for your convenience.
- Close the cap of the bottle and mix the oils well.
- Then keep the bottle in cool and dry place.
- Place the diffuser cap at the top of the bottle.
- Press the button to have its fumes out whenever you need.

Recipe no. 20

Ingredients:

- Rosemary oil 2 teaspoon
- Coconut oil 3 teaspoon
- Grapefruit oil 4 drops
- Celery seed oil 4 drops
- Black pepper oil 2 drops

Method:

- Take a small container and add all the ingredients that have been mentioned above.
- Beware that you are taking the right quantity just according to what have been mentioned in the ingredients above.
- Make the cap of the bottle closed and mix the oils well so that they can become smooth in consistency.
- Leave the bottle for about 3 days in a dry place or you can also place it in the sun for 3 to 3 hours daily so that the body spray can be enriched.
- Place the diffuser cap at the top of the bottle.
- Press the button to have its fumes out whenever you need.

10 spring and summer essential oil diffuser recipes

Recipe no. 1

Ingredients:

Jojoba oil 4 drops

Almond oil 4 drops

Poppy seeds 2 teaspoon

Method:

- Mix all ingredients.
- Leave in dry place for about two days.
- Place the diffuser cap at the top of the bottle.
- Press the button to have its fumes out whenever you need.

Recipe no. 2

Ingredients:

Honey 4 drops

Jojoba oil 4 drops

Carrot oil 4 drops

Orange peel essential oil 2 drops

Method:

- Combine all ingredients.
- Leave in dry place for about two days.
- Place the diffuser cap at the top of the bottle.
- Press the button to have its fumes out whenever you need.

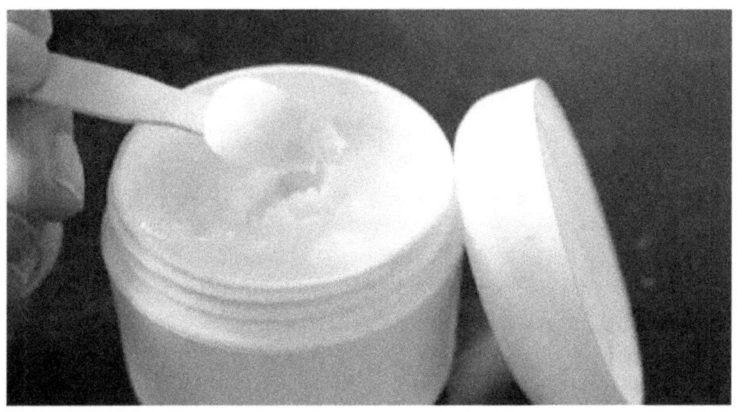

Recipe no. 3

Ingredients:

Jojoba oil 4 drops

Turmeric powder 1 teaspoon

Hazel drops 1 teaspoon

Method:

- Combine all ingredients.

- Then keep the bottle in cool and dry place.

- Place the diffuser cap at the top of the bottle.

- Press the button to have its fumes out whenever you need.

Recipe no. 4

Ingredients:

Lemon essential oil 4 drops

Almond oil 2 drops

Strawberry essential oil 2 drops

Method:

- Combine all ingredients.
- Then keep the bottle in cool and dry place.
- Place the diffuser cap at the top of the bottle.
- Press the button to have its fumes out whenever you need.

Recipe no. 5

Ingredients:

- Rose essential oil 3 drops

- Lemon oil 3 drops

Method:

- Take a small bottle or container and add all the ingredients that have been mentioned in the above-mentioned list for your convenience.

- Then keep the bottle in cool and dry place.

- Place the diffuser cap at the top of the bottle.

- Press the button to have its fumes out whenever you need.

Recipe no. 6

Ingredients:

Tea tree oil 2 teaspoon

Peppermint oil 1 teaspoon

Almond oil 4 drops

Method:

- Combine all ingredients.
- Then keep the bottle in cool and dry place.
- Place the diffuser cap at the top of the bottle.
- Press the button to have its fumes out whenever you need.

Recipe no. 7

Ingredients:

- Rose essential oil 3 drops
- Jasmine essential oil 3 drops
- Cumin oil 3 drops
- Lemon oil 3 drops
- Savory oil 3 drops

Method:

- Take a small bottle or container and add all the ingredients that have been mentioned in the above-mentioned list for your convenience.
- Close the bottle's cap tightly so that no air can enter inside and mix all the mixtures well so that you can get the desired consistency out of it without any ambiguity on your way.
- Then keep the bottle in cool and dry place.
- Place the diffuser cap at the top of the bottle.
- Press the button to have its fumes out whenever you need.

Recipe no. 8

Ingredients:

Jojoba oil 4 drops

Raspberry oil 2 teaspoon

Method:

- Combine all ingredients.

- Then keep the bottle in cool and dry place.

- Place the diffuser cap at the top of the bottle.

- Press the button to have its fumes out whenever you need.

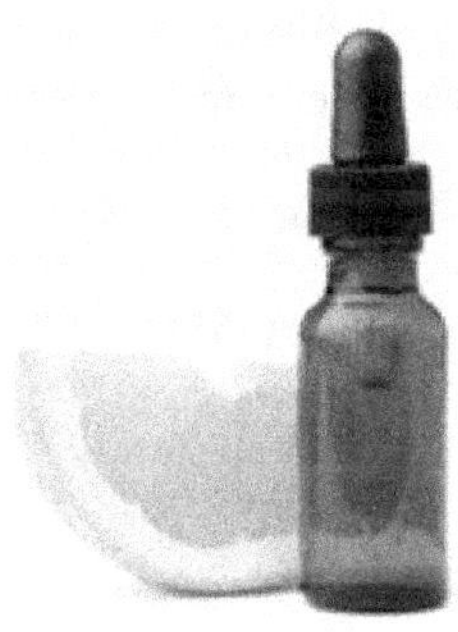

Recipe no. 9

Ingredients:

- Rose essential oil 3 drops
- Jasmine essential oil 3 drops
- Cumin oil 3 drops
- Lemon oil 3 drops
- Savory oil 3 drops

Method:

- Take a small bottle or container and add all the ingredients above.
- Close the bottle's cap tightly so that no air can enter inside and mix all the mixtures well so that you can get the desired consistency out of it without any ambiguity on your way.
- Then keep the bottle in cool and dry place.
- Place the diffuser cap at the top of the bottle.
- Press the button to have its fumes out whenever you need.

Recipe no. 10

Ingredients:

Jojoba oil 3 drops

Hazel 1 teaspoon

Almond oil 4 drops

Raspberry essential oil

Method:

- Combine all ingredients.

- Then keep the bottle in cool and dry place.

- Place the diffuser cap at the top of the bottle.

- Press the button to have its fumes out whenever you need.

Chapter 11 – Amazing Essential Oil Diffusers for Sleep

There are lots of essential oils that can help you to relieve the symptoms of stress, anxiety and depression and enjoy a sound sleep. You can treat your anxiety with the use of some scented essential oils. A right scent will make you happy; therefore, you should select a scent carefully. Following are some essential oils that can help you to get rid of tension and depression:

- **Basil Essential Oil:** It can enhance your mood and work to remove emotions of anxiety, fatigue and depress.

- **Clary Safe Essential Oil:** It is an excellent essential oil to get rid of insomnia, tension, anxiety, and depression.

- **Frankincense:** If you are suffering from stress, anxiety, fear and tension, then you should use this essential oil to slow down these emotions.

- **Geranium Essential Oil:** It may reduce your stress and depression because it naturally works to enhance the spirit and release the negative emotions out.

- **Jasmine Essential Oil:** It is a relaxing and an antispasmodic essential oil with mood-lifting properties.

- **Lemon Essential Oil:** The refreshing scent of the lemon essential oil can enhance your mood. It enables you to fight with the stress, negative emotions, and depression.

- **Mandarin Essential Oil:** The antispasmodic properties help you to uplift the spirit.

- **Marjoram:** If you are feeling grief, fear, rejection, anxiety, and loneliness, then this is an excellent essential oil to enhance your mood.

- **Wild Orange:** It is good to increase your energy and enhance your mood. It is excellent to relieve the feelings of anger, irritation, and nervousness.

- **Palmarosa:** It is excellent for the treatment of nervous tension and anxiety.

- **Rose:** It can stimulate the sense of well-being by treating tension and nervousness.

- **Roman Chamomile:** It is ideal to relax your body and mind. It is an ultimate treatment for the depression and stress.

- **Sandalwood:** Its scent has magical properties to relieve tension and stress.

- **Ylang-Ylang:** The relaxing scent of ylang-ylang is equally good to energize both men and women. The scent of this essential oil can increase your confidence and treat depression, insomnia, and stress.

BLENDS
for sleep!

6 DROPS RUTAVALA

4 DROPS LAVENDER
4 DROPS PEACE & CALMING

4 DROPS LAVENDER
3 DROPS BERGAMOT

4 DROPS FRANKINCENSE
3 DROPS VETIVER

2 DROPS LAVENDER
2 DROPS CEDARWOOD
2 DROPS PEACE & CALMING

3 DROPS LAVENDER
3 DROPS ROMAN CHAMOMILE
1 DROP VETIVER

2 DROPS LAVENDER
2 DROPS VETIVER
2 DROPS VALERIAN
2 DROPS ORANGE

4 DROPS LAVENDER
1 DROP BERGAMOT
1 DROP PATCHOULI
1 DROP YLANG YLANG

Essential Oils for Loneliness

Isolation and loneliness are not good for anyone because it can harm you because during isolation, your mind filled with lots of negative thoughts and emotions. You prefer to live in isolation, but during the adverse times, it is important to take the help of your friends and love. The Ayurveda offers the best solution and it is meditation. You can talk to God during medication and offer a small prayer to comfort yourself. This will bring a great difference in your condition. There are some essential oils that will give you the energy to fight with the loneliness and support your mind.

Special Blend for Loneliness

If you are feeling lonely, then try this blend to get power for your mind and body:

- Rose oil

- Chamomile oil

- Frankincense oil

- Clary sages oil

- Bergamot oil

Take 1 to 2 drops of the oils and add into your bathtub to take a bath. You need to use a diffuser to reduce the intensity of the oils. You can use olive oil or almond oil as a carrier oil to defuse the blend. It will be good to apply this blend on your handkerchief and keep it with you to get energy and power to fight lonesomeness.

Note: The helichrysum and palo santo essential oils are also good to treat loneliness.

Chapter 12 – Get Rid of Stress and Anxiety with Essential Oil Diffusers

If you are dealing with anxious feelings, then it is important to use essential oils because these are better to use as compared to medicines. Following are some essential oils that you can use to treat your anxiety:

Balance Essential Oil

This essential oil is a blend of rosewood, blue tansy, spruce, and frankincense. It is an ideal essential oil to treat your anxiety. You can get a feeling of calmness with the use of this oil. It is a natural remedy used to calm down your nerves and promote the relaxation. The chamomile is used to soothe your nerves. The Frankincense can promote your relaxation and relieve the feelings of sorrow.

Lavender Essential Oil

If you are dealing with anxiousness, then you can try the lavender essential oil. Its scent is really calm and attractive, and you can use it in the water while taking a bath. You can also add it few drops in the deodorant to make it relaxing. There is a number of scientific proves that the lavender can reduce the anxiety and enhance the mood of patients.

Wild Orange Essential Oils

Wild orange essential oil is a great choice to reduce anxiety and boost your mood. It can increase your happiness and well-being. It is not good to eat any essential oil, but you can add a few drops of orange essential oils in your recipe to enhance citrus flavor.

Serenity Essential Oil

Serenity is a useful essential oil prepared to treat your anxiety. You can combine this essential oil with the lavender, sweet marjoram, ylang-ylang, sandalwood, and vanilla. These all oils have excellent properties, and you can enjoy a massage of these oils to promote sleep. The ylang-ylang is really beneficial for your central nervous system. The serenity can be applied topically or you may diffuse it in the air. You can apply it to the bottom of your feet before going to bed to enjoy a deep and relaxing sleep.

Bergamot Essential Oil

The bergamot is used to relieve the tension and stress, and it can also be used to improve the health of your skin. It features citrus scent and you can use it to enhance your mood. The bergamot can promote the relaxation by reducing the feelings of anxiousness. It is the best essential oil to apply to the skin or diffuse in the air to treating the tension and promote a good sleep. In order to enhance the benefits of essential oils, it will be good to use magnesium supplement to overcome your anxious feelings.

Grounding Blend

It is a useful blend of howood, spruce, frankincense and chamomile. If you are suffering from anxiety and tension, then this blend will really help you. It can promote the feelings of calmness and reduce your stress.

Application:

The grounding blend can be applied to your feet on a regular basis. You can also massage it over the back of your neck, heart and the wrists get better results.

Apply on the wrists and rub them together and inhale. You can mix this oil with a calming blend to increase its benefits.

Respiratory Blend

It is a versatile blend used for all respiratory issues. It is a combination of peppermint, lemon, ravensara lead, melaleuca and Cardamom seeds. It will help you to calm down your brain during anxiety.

Application:

Apply a few drops on your chest to relax your nerves and open your airways for relaxed breathing.

Frankincense

It is a king of essential oils that is why it is really valuable to slow down the fear, anxiety and tension. If you are suffering from stressful feelings, then it is an excellent choice for you. It can help you to combat the feelings of fear and anxiety.

Directions:

It is a great oil for regular use because it can promote your cellular balance. It can reduce feelings of anxiety, so use it in the diffuse state. You can inhale it, or massage your feet and back with a few drops of oil. Blend of lavender oil and wild orange can help you to get rid of anxiety.

Try a Joyful Blend

The smell of this oil will be great to treat the feelings of anxiety and tensions. It can treat anxiety and depression at the same time. The blend contains lavender, tangerine, elemi, lemon, Melissa, ylang-ylang, sandalwood, and osmanthus.

Directions:

You can apply it on your heart, bones, behind the ear, neck, forehead and wrists to reduce stress. Its regular application will help you to calm your mind and get rid of tensions.

Lemon Essential Oil

It is a versatile oil with lots of benefits because of its properties. The lemon oil is excellent to uplift your mood, revive your stressful feelings, and stimulate your feelings. The lemon enhances the sense of security and trust. It can help you to remove confusions and tensions. It can clear the obstacles and improve your feelings.

Directions:

You can use it on a regular basis in water. Just add 1 drop of essential oil in a glass of water and then use it for the whole day.

Calming Blend

If you want to promote relaxed feelings, then this blend is excellent for you. It can control your anger and promote good health with calmness. The blend contains sweet marjoram, lavender, ylang-ylang, roman chamomile, sandalwood, and vanilla bean.

Direction:

Use almost 5 drops of this blend in the hot water for relaxation. You can also apply it on the back of your neck and inhale it through a diffuser. Some drops should be applied to the bottoms of your feet before going to sleep. Awesome smell can leave excellent effects on your nerves.

Patchouli Essential Oil

It is a special oil to harmonize your mind and keep it stable without any tension. It can reduce the negative thoughts by relieving the depression and increase the joy in your life. You can recover from tension, stress and tiredness of mind.

Direction:

You can apply a diffused form of this oil to the base of your skull. Inhale the aroma of the oil to calm your fortitude and reduce disorganized thoughts.

Woody Diffuser for Calming Effects

Cypress oil: 2 drops

White first oil: 2 drops

Wintergreen oil: 2 drops

Spiced Chai

Cardamom oil: 3 drops

Cassia oil: 2 drops

Clove oil: 2 drops

Ginger oil: 1 drop

Enjoy Autumn Smell

Wild orange oil: 3 drops

Cinnamon bark oil: 2 drops

Clove oil: 1 drop

Calming Effects

Frankincense oil: 3 drops

White fir oil: 2 drops

Cedarwood oil: 1 drop

Boost Immunity

Rosemary oil: 1 drop

Clove oil: 1 drop

Cinnamon bark oil: 1 drop

Eucalyptus oil: 1 drop

Wild orange oil: 1 drop

Stress Buster Blend

Frankincense oil: 2 drops

Bergamot oil: 2 drops

Enhance Sleep

Lavender oil: 2 drops

Chamomile oil: 2 drops

Vetiver essential oil: 2 drops

Chapter 13 – Essential Oil Diffusers to Enhance Happiness

Everyone has its own reasons to become happy, but if you want to increase your joy, then you should use some essential oils. These oils can help you to enhance the joy in your life. There are lots of uses of these essential oils, such as you can increase your joy and happiness of your party by diffusing few oils. You can also memorize the days of winter holidays by using Cinnamon, Ginger, and a little Orange essential oil. Put a few drops of these oils in the evaporator to increase the happiness. The blend of various oils will be a unique way to enhance your mood. Some blends of essential oils help women to stabilize their hormones. The blend will only help women without affecting the hormonal balance of another person in the house. Following are some essential oils that will help you to increase your happiness.

Bergamot Essential Oil

The fresh, citrus oil and refreshing scent of the essential oils can uplift your mood. The aroma of this oil will help you to feel bright, happy and energized. It is excellent for your healthy skin and improve good health. It is useful for its antiseptic properties, particularly for the skin that is prone to acne. It is useful for eczema and other conditions that can increase stress.

Geranium Essential Oil

This is an excellent essential oil to harmonize, comfort, calm and balance your mood. It can uplift your mood and strengthen your mind to get rid of tensions and anxiety. It is a wonderful oil for skin care and treat menopause condition as well. The oil is equally good to use for a healthy and excellent skin. If you have dry and oily skin, you can use it because of its antiseptic and anti-inflammatory properties. It can heal the reasons of tension and uplift your mood.

Enhance Happiness

Wild orange: 2 drops

Wintergreen oil: 2 drops

Boost Your Mood

Wild orange oil: 2 drops

Frankincense oil: 2 drops

Cinnamon oil: 2 drops

Chillout Essential Oil

Vetiver essential oil: 2 drops

Cedarwood essential oil: 2 drops

Happy Diffuser Oil

Wild orange: 2 drops

White fir: 2 drops

Wintergreen: 1 drop

Chapter 14 – Essential Oil Diffusers to Manage Anger

There are lots of essential oils that can help you to relax. The strong aroma of these oils will relax your nerves and help you to control negative emotions. Following are some essential oils that are really beneficial for your health:

Peace and Calming Blend

You can prepare a blend of orange, tangerine, ylang-ylang, blue tansy and patchouli because this blend is excellent to manage your anger. It can promote the feelings of peace and reduce your stress level.

Directions:

If you want to treat your anger, then you should consider this blend because the massage of this oil will help you to manage anger. Use it in a diffused state and promote peace and calmness. Add a drop of oil in your bath water, or you can use it as a perfume as well.

Ylang Ylang

It is an excellent essential oil used in a diffused form to treat anger. The properties of this special essential oil will help you to reduce anxiety, blood pressure, frustration and much more.

Directions:

If you want to take the benefits of this essential oil, then apply it on your feet in a diffused form. You can also rub it on your spin on your lower back to get rid of anger.

Roman Chamomile Essential Oil

If an angry outburst is an important part of your conversation, then you should try this essential oil. This oil has magical properties to treat allergy, cleanse your blood, calm your sorrow and grieves.

Directions:

You can apply this essential oil on your throat in a diffused form. It will help you to stabilize your anger and bring your emotions to a balance.

Lavender Essential Oil

The lavender is famous for its soothing and calming properties because after its application, you can feel relaxed. It can treat allergies, digestion problems; reduce nausea and many other problems. Its regular massage will promote your good health and enhance your mood.

Directions:

The lavender can be inhaled from the bottle, or you can rub the back of your neck after taking this oil on your hands. It will help you to reduce stress and tension. The oil has excellent properties to diffuse your anger.

Geranium Essential Oil

This is an excellent essential oil, and you should include it in your daily routine. The essential oil is excellent to make your skin beautiful and support your circulatory and nervous system. It is excellent to invigorate your body tissues.

Directions:

You can use this oil to promote brain health, and it is quite easy to use because it is good to inhale it directly. Few drops of diffused geranium essential oil can be rubbed on your neck to get rid of anger.

Sandalwood Essential Oil

The sandalwood essential oil can treat your emotional issues, relieve stress and unwind the tensions. Aloes are its other name, and you can rub your backbone, wrist, and neck with the help of diffused sandalwood essential oil. This oil is really good for your skin. After its frequent use, you can be able to get rid of all tensions and anger emotions.

Blue Tansy Essential Oil

It has slightly sweet aroma and used to manage anger. If you are suffering from anger and other negative emotions, then use this essential oil because it has lots of benefits. The famous species of tansy plants are Moroccan and Chamomile.

Directions:

- Take a few drops of diffused essential oil, and apply it on your feet. It can calm your mind and alleviate the negative emotions.

- You can also add a few drops in your bath to promote the feelings of relaxation.

Soothing Blends:

Following are some blends that will help you to promote the feelings of relaxation and enhance your mood:

Blend 01:

- 1 drop Rose

- 3 drops Orange

- 1 drop Vetiver

Mix all these essential oils and pour it in the water before taking a bath. It will help you to reduce anger.

Blend 02:

- 3 drops Bergamot

- 1 drop Ylang Ylang

- 1 drop Jasmine

Add this blend to your bath water and take a bath with it to gradually reduce your anger.

Blend 03:

- 1 drop Roman Chamomile

- 2 drops Bergamot

- 2 Drops Orange Essential Oil

Take a relaxing bath after adding this blend in a bucket of water, and get the benefits of this bath.

Blend 04:

- 3 drops of Orange Essential Oil

- 2 drops of Patchouli Oil

This will be the relaxing blend for to manage your anger. Include it in a bucket of water to take a bath or add it in a diffuser to keep it in your room

Tips to Diffuse Your Blend

You can increase the amount of blend by adding your oil in a dark colored bottle made of glass and then roll the bottle between your hands. You can add a diffuser like olive oil to diffuse the blend and use this blend in your bath water.

Carrier Oils

The carrier oils are often used as a diffuser to diffuse the intensity of carrier oils. You can mix these oils with essential oils to take aromatherapy. Following are some famous and frequently used carrier oils:

- Sweet almond oil

- Olive oil

- Sunflower oil

In short, the seed, vegetable, and nut oils can be used to dilute the concentrated essential oils.

Rose Essential Oils

The rose essential oils are famous for its properties because it can be used as an antidepressant, antiseptic, antispasmodic, hepatic, uterine, stomachic, etc. The rose essential oil works well to alleviate stress, mental tension, depression, nervous ailments and various other problems. If you want to get rid of anger and mental stress, then use rose essential oil to manage this situation.

Palo Santo Essential Oil

The palo santo essential oil is used to manage anger because its scent can keep your mind free from worries and tensions. Its anti-inflammatory properties can help you to avoid cancer as well. The regular use of this oil will help you to manage anger and stress.

Diffuser

- 5 drops Cedarwood Atlas

- 4 drops Palo Santo

- 1 drop Patchouli

- 5 drops of Bergamot

Bug Repellent Diffuser of Essential Oil

Lemongrass oil: 1 drop

Thyme oil: 1 drop

Eucalyptus oil: 1 drop

Basil oil: 1 drop

Chapter 15 – Increase Your Confidence with Essential Oil Diffusers

There are lots of essential oils that are used during performing religious traditions. The exotic fragrance and purities of the essential oil can improve your mood. There are a number of essential oils that can be used to increase self-confidence.

Cypress Essential Oil

The cypress essential oil is famous for its properties because it can help you to treat lots of problems. It can help you to extricate stuck emotions. If you are feeling any tension and want to ignore everything, then push things aside and shove negative emotions. The negative emotions make it really hard to feel relaxed and the cypress can help you to bring an accurate balance to your mind and spirit. You can get rid of fear and treat your negative emotions with the help of cypress essential oil.

Directions:

You can use it in diluted form and then massage several locations of your body. You should consider the vita flex points to get optimum benefits.

Peppermint Essential Oils

If you want to enhance your energy and confidence, then the peppermint essential oil will be an excellent drug for you. There is no need to drink caffeine because the essential oil can increase your energy levels. The peppermint oil trickles the freshness and improves your mental health. It can keep you alert and enables you to tackle each task in a better way.

Directions:

Peppermint essential oil can uplift your mood and confidence. You can include a few drops of peppermint oil in your bath water to keep your mind fresh. It will reduce tension, anxiety and enhance the feelings of calmness. In the absence of tension and anxiety, you can perform in a better way.

Sandalwood Essential Oil

If you have dry or irritated skin, then you may feel low in the public places because a smooth and beautiful skin can boost your confidence. With dull and dry skin, you will only think about the negative views of people about you. If you want a glowing and healthy skin, then you should add a few drops of sandalwood essential oil in your body lotion. It will make your skin healthy and increase its glow. When you feel good in your own skin, your self-confidence will be at a higher level.

Bergamot Essential Oil

The bergamot essential oil is an excellent addition to your daily routine because it can improve the health of your skin. It is often used in the production of perfumes and has amazing healing powers. This oil is equally good for your brain because it can cure your stress, tension, and anger in a better way. If you want to increase your self-confidence, you should reduce your stress, anxiety, and tension. The Bergamot essential oil will play an important role in this.

Rosemary Essential Oil

If you want to boost your confidence, then you should focus on your personal improvement. The rosemary essential oil will increase the shine and smooth texture of your hair. Just add five drops of rosemary oil in the bottle of shampoo. It will make your hair silky and keep your scalp free from dandruff. If you are suffering from migraines, then instead of using tablets, try this oil. Use a drop of this oil and massage on your wrists. Take q few deep breaths and feel the calm sensation.

Tea Tree Essential Oil

If you are feeling any problem just because of virus and bacteria around you, then you should use tea tree oil. The oil will serve as a body bouncer and improve the immune system of your body in a natural way. It will save your money because after using this, there is no need to use expensive treatments. You can pamper your skin with the help of this oil because it may reduce the acne from your skin. Tea tree oil will be an ultimate solution of your all problems. Take a bath by adding a few drops of tea tree essential oils in water.

Chamomile Essential Oil

It is quite surprising to know that the chamomile is an excellent mood booster. If you are feeling burdened and want to get rid of these feelings, then use this oil. Just add a few drops of chamomile oil in the boiling water, and take a bath to see its magic.

Ylang-Ylang Essential Oil

If you have ylang-ylang essential oil, then you can turn your own bathroom into a spa by adding a few drops of this oil in water. This will help you to control your emotions, and you may feel relaxed. This essential oil is available in a small bottle, and you can use it in different ways. If you don't want to take a bath, then you can add a few drops in a very small bottle and spray this water on your face. It will enhance the feelings of calmness and relaxation. This is an excellent mood booster and increases your self-confidence as well.

There are lots of powerful essential oils that can increase your self-confidence and enhance your mood. You can inhale these oils or take a bath by adding a few drops. If you want to enjoy enough benefits of essential oils, then find the right oil for you to restore your energy. It will increase your self-confidence by boosting your mood.

Diffuser to Increase Your Alertness

Wild orange oil: 2 drops

Peppermint oil: 2 drops

Fresh Diffuser of Essential Oil

Lavender oil: 2 drops

Lemon oil: 2 drops

Rosemary oil: 2 drops

Odor Eliminator

Lemon oil: 2 drops

Melaleuca oil: 1 drop

Cilantro oil: 1 drop

Lime oil: 1 drop

Seasonal Diffuser

Lavender oil: 2 drops

Lemon oil: 2 drops

Peppermint oil: 2 drops

Citrus Explosion Oil

Lemon oil: 1 drop

Wild orange oil: 2 drops

Lime oil: 1 drop

Grapefruit oil: 1 drop

Deep Breath Essential Oil Diffusers

Bergamot oil: 1 drop

Patchouli oil: 1 drop

Ylang ylang oil: 1 drop

Respiratory Blend

Lemon oil: 1 drop

Eucalyptus oil: 1 drop

Peppermint oil: 2 drops

Rosemary oil: 1 drop

Flower Garden Diffuser

Lavender oil: 2 drops

Geranium oil: 1 drop

Roman Chamomile oil: 2 drops

Precautionary Tips for Essential Oil

It is really good to use essential oils, but you have to consider safety and effectiveness. Following are some general guideline and precautions that will help you:

- You need to keep essential oils away from the reach of children and pets.

- The essential oils with high menthol like peppermint should not be used on the throat and neck of the children under 30 months.

- The essential oils can't dilute in the water; therefore, you can mix them in the vegetable oil to dissolve in water.

- The oils are available in the concentrated state; therefore, you should use them in diluted form. The concentrated oil should not come in contact with the sensitive skin areas.

- Undiluted oils should not be directly poured into the bath water.

- If you have sensitive skin, then the oil should not be applied directly on the skin. Dilute it with a carrier oil and then apply to the neat and clean soles of the feet.

- If you have allergies, then you should be careful while using essential oils. The sole of your feet is the least sensitive area, and you can apply oil on the sole.

- Some essential oils have strong caustic properties; dilute these essential oils before using them.

- Some citrus essential like orange, lemon and bergamot and petitgrain should not be applied directly on the skin if you have to go out. These oils are phototoxic and you need to avoid direct sunlight for almost 48hours.

- Before trying any kind of essential oil, you need to do a patch test of the diluted oil to know if it is irritating you.

- A number of essential oils are not good to ingest; therefore, you have to be careful. Properly know the properties of the essential oils before ingesting them. It is good to take the advice of your health care advisor before consuming any oil.

- If you have sensitive skin, heart and kidney problems, asthma, and other serious medical conditions, then you should consult your doctor for the safety of any essential oil for you.

- The properties of essential oil can't be judged on the basis of the properties of its plants.

- Keep the essential oils away from heat, flame, and all ignition sources.

- You need to be careful while applying essential oils on the skin because some personal care products may contain synthetic and petrochemicals. These can penetrate and remain in the skin and fatty tissues for various days. The essential oils can react with these chemicals to cause irritation, nausea, and other displeasures.

- There can be a strong reaction of essential oils on the body because of the chemicals in food, water, and the environment. If your skin gets any reaction, then stop the use of essential oil and start internal cleansing before resuming to the regular routine. You can increase the water intake to reduce any adverse reaction.

Precautions for An Accident with Essential Oils

If an essential oil falls into your eyes accidentally, the immediately flush it with cold milk or vegetable oil to dilute the oil. If you still feel any stinging, you can consult a doctor immediately.

You can use cream or vegetable oil to remove the additional essential oils from your skin. Use soap and warm water to remove additional oil from the skin.

If you ingest any essential oil accidently, then you can call national poison control center for assistance.

Conclusion

There you have it, everything you need to know to get well versed in the use of essential oils. With this book, you will know not only what kind of oils to use for certain ailments, but you will also know which blends to make and how to administer for the greatest results.

Discover your perfect method, combine that with your favorite blends, and reap the excellent benefits that are sure to follow. In no time at all you will know just what to do with any ailment that arises, no matter what time of the day it is.

I hope this book is able to show you how you can treat any ailment naturally, and you can do it your way. No strict rules, no crazy side effects to worry about, and absolutely none of that medicinal smell that you don't want on you or your children.

Natural remedies are by far the best way to go, and when you know what you are doing, you have the very key you need to make it happen. That is what this book aims to do, and that is exactly what you will be able by the time you have reached this point.

I hope you now feel the confidence I know you should have, and that you are able to treat and prevent a variety of ailments that arise in day to day living. These treatments are the best of the best. They have been around for thousands of years for a reason... they work!

Forget the stress that comes from going to the store and standing in the medication aisle for hours, trying to decide which one is best for you. Now, you can treat anything you can think of naturally, and naturally you can do it whenever you please.

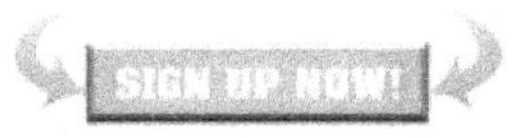

OR Go to this URL

http://zbit.ly/1WBb1Ek